1998

HEADLINE SERIES

No. 309   FOREIGN POLICY ASSOCIATION   Winter

Microbes Versus Mankind:
The Coming Plague

by Laurie Garrett

Cover Design: Ed Bohon $5.95

The Author

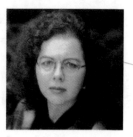

LAURIE GARRETT is a health and science writer for *Newsday*. A contributing author to *AIDS in the World*, edited by Jonathan Mann, she was formerly a science correspondent for National Public Radio and has written for *The Washington Post Magazine*, the *Los Angeles Times*, and *Omni*, among many other publications. Garrett researched *The Coming Plague* as a fellow at the Harvard School of Public Health.

The Foreign Policy Association

The Foreign Policy Association is a private, nonprofit, nonpartisan educational organization. Its purpose is to stimulate wider interest and more effective participation in, and greater understanding of, world affairs among American citizens. Among its activities is the continuous publication, dating from 1935, of the HEADLINE SERIES. The author is responsible for factual accuracy and for the views expressed. FPA itself takes no position on issues of U.S. foreign policy.

HEADLINE SERIES (ISSN 0017-8780) is published four times a year, Spring, Summer, Fall and Winter, by the Foreign Policy Association, Inc., 470 Park Avenue So., New York, N.Y. 10016. Chairman, Paul B. Ford; President, Noel V. Lateef; Editor in Chief, Nancy Hoepli-Phalon; Senior Editors, Ann R. Monjo and K.M. Rohan; Associate Editor, June Lee. Subscription rates, $20.00 for 4 issues; $35.00 for 8 issues; $50.00 for 12 issues. Single copy price $5.95; double issue $11.25. Discount 25% on 10 to 99 copies; 30% on 100 to 499; 35% on 500 and over. Payment must accompany all orders. Postage and handling: $2.50 for first copy; $.50 each additional copy. Second-class postage paid at New York, N.Y., and additional mailing offices. POSTMASTER: Send address changes to HEADLINE SERIES, Foreign Policy Association, 470 Park Avenue So., New York, N.Y. 10016. Copyright 1996 by Foreign Policy Association, Inc. Design by K.M. Rohan. Printed at Science Press, Ephrata, Pennsylvania. Winter 1994. Published April 1996.

Library of Congress Catalog Card No. 96-84227
ISBN 0-87124-169-2

Introduction

I N 1981 Dr. Richard Krause of the U.S. National Institutes of Health published a provocative book entitled *The Restless Tide: The Persistent Challenge of the Microbial World,* which argued that diseases long thought to have been defeated could return to endanger the American people. In hearings a year later before the U.S. Congress, Krause was asked, "Why do we have so many new infectious diseases?"

"Nothing new has happened," Krause replied. "Plagues are as certain as death and taxes."

University of Chicago historian William McNeill outlined the reasons *Homo sapiens* had been vulnerable to microbial assaults over the millennia. He saw each catastrophic epidemic event in human history as the ironic result of humanity's steps forward. As humans improve their lots, McNeill warned, they actually *increase* their vulnerability to disease.

"It is, I think, worthwhile being conscious of the limits upon our powers," McNeill said. "It is worth keeping in mind that the more we win, the more we drive infections to the margins of human experience, the more we clear a path for possible catastrophic infection. We'll never escape the limits of the ecosys-

---

The selections that constitute this issue of the HEADLINE SERIES have been excerpted by K. M. Rohan from a much larger work, *The Coming Plague,* by Laurie Garrett (Farrar, Straus & Giroux, 1994).

tem. We are caught in the food chain, whether we like it or not, eating and being eaten."

Over the last five years, scientists have voiced concern that HIV, far from representing a public-health aberration, may be a sign of things to come. They warn that humanity has learned little about preparedness and response to new microbes, despite the blatant tragedy of AIDS. And they call for recognition of the ways in which changes at the micro level of the environment of any nation can affect life at the global, macro level.

Humanity's ancient enemies are, after all, microbes. They didn't go away just because science invented drugs, antibiotics and vaccines (with the notable exception of smallpox). They didn't disappear from the planet when Americans and Europeans cleaned up their towns and cities in the postindustrial era. And they certainly won't become extinct simply because human beings choose to ignore their existence.

In this book I explore the recent history of disease emergence, examining in roughly chronological order examples that highlight reasons for microbial epidemics and the ways humans respond. The book also examines the biology of evolution at the microbial level, looking closely at ways in which disease agents and their vectors are adapting to counter the defensive weapons used to protect human beings. In addition, it looks at means by which humans are actually aiding and abetting the microbes through ill-planned development schemes, misguided medicine, errant public health, and shortsighted political action/inaction.

What is required, overall, is a new paradigm in the way people think about disease. Rather than a view that sees humanity's relationship to the microbes as a historically linear one, tending over the centuries toward ever-decreasing risk to humans, a far more challenging perspective must be sought. As Harvard University's Dick Levins puts it, "we must embrace complexity, seek ways to describe and comprehend an ever-changing ecology we cannot see, but, nonetheless, by which we are constantly affected."

1

Battles with Microbes:
Winner and Loser

IMBUED with profound optimism, coupled with the post-
World War II American "can do" attitude, the world's
public-health community mounted two ambitious campaigns to
eradicate microbes from the planet. One effort would succeed,
becoming the greatest triumph of modern public health. The
other would fail so miserably that the targeted microbes would
increase both in numbers and in virulence, and the *Homo sapiens* death toll would soar.

Humanity's great success story would be smallpox.

In 1958 the Soviet Union went before the World Health
Assembly—the legislative body of the World Health Organization (WHO) in Geneva, Switzerland—to request an international campaign for the elimination of smallpox, winning
virtually universal support.

Historically, smallpox had proven a particularly vicious killer.
In A.D. 165, the Roman Empire was devastated by an epidemic
now believed to have been smallpox. The pestilence raged for

15 years, claiming victims in all social strata in such high numbers that some parts of the Roman Empire lost 25 to 35 percent of their people. It is believed that the virus struck a completely nonimmune population, having first appeared in Asia some 100 years earlier.

Over subsequent centuries equally devastating pandemics of the viral disease claimed millions of lives in China, Japan, the Roman Empire, Europe and the Americas. Smallpox, together with measles, tuberculosis and influenza, claimed an estimated 56 million Amerindian lives during the initial years of the Spanish conquest.

By 1958, when the Soviets called for global eradication, smallpox was killing 2 million people a year, and cases could be found in 33 countries.

Both the historic devastation and the widespread rates of contemporary infection seemed to argue for skepticism about smallpox eradication.

On the other hand, several aspects of the biology of smallpox gave cause for optimism. Foremost was the existence of an extremely effective vaccine that, in various forms, had been in use since 1796. In modern times the cowpox vaccine, made from the bovine form of the virus, had been perfected, making it over 99 percent effective, with virtually no side effects. Smallpox was also easy to diagnose, and cases of the disease could readily be spotted by people with no professional training. During severe illness, grotesque bulbous inflammations formed on the individual's face and skin. The distinct poxing, once healed, left visible scars anybody could recognize.

Because the virus was spread directly from person to person there were no troublesome vectors to control, such as mosquitoes, rats, ticks, or fleas. And the very thing that made smallpox so terrifying—its rapid lethality—also rendered it controllable because the viruses multiplied and spread so quickly that most people were infectious for only four or five days and their debilitation was so great that they could not walk about and infect large numbers of people.

Though eradication would require over 250 million vaccine

doses per year and a worldwide effort to reach all citizens at risk for smallpox—even those in the midst of wars, social tyranny, famine, or disaster—the program began amid optimism in 1967 under the leadership of American physician Donald "D. A." Henderson.

Nations of the Northern Hemisphere and Latin America were already well on their way to smallpox eradication in 1967, but the disease was firmly in place in many parts of Africa and Asia, where religion often proved a major barrier to vaccination.

Before the campaign began, researchers scoured pilot-project areas to see how accurately smallpox cases were reported. Their conclusion was that an astonishing 95 percent of all cases of the disease were never reported to national or international public-health authorities. The reasons for such dramatic underreporting were numerous: local authorities feared being penalized if higher-ups learned that epidemics had occurred in their jurisdictions; in some areas the disease was simply accepted as a fact of life; outbreaks tended to occur in confined areas and could easily be missed by quick national surveys; during centuries of colonialism, people's homes were often burned if smallpox was found in a family member, so people in former colonies naturally concluded it was best not to inform authorities.

WHO Team on the Attack

Ultimately, Henderson's team at WHO devised a smallpox plan of attack that boldly confronted these issues by dispersing dozens of skilled tropical-disease experts all over the world in search of small outbreaks of the virus. Once such an outbreak was identified, local government was mobilized and residents of the area were vaccinated. Inoculation was occasionally carried out forcibly; in some instances people's homes were invaded and local police assisted the inoculators.

Because both superpowers (the United States and the U.S.S.R.) wholeheartedly supported the campaign, few governments resisted public-health efforts that often took on military overtones. The WHO teams braved civil wars, floods, religious battles, and a variety of geographic and logistic problems to accomplish their task.

In 1972 Don Francis had just barely completed his pediatrics residency at Los Angeles County Hospital and signed on with the U.S. Centers for Disease Control and Prevention (CDC) in Atlanta, Georgia, when smallpox broke out in Kosovo, Yugoslavia. The young doctor was just setting up a CDC disease-surveillance office in Oregon when Atlanta called, ordering him to go to Belgrade, Yugoslavia. Seven hours later he was in Washington, D.C., getting a briefing and cases of vaccination equipment. Before midnight he was asleep on a jet flying somewhere over the Atlantic, and in the morning he hit the ground running in Belgrade.

A few weeks later, the Yugoslavia outbreak safely contained, Francis was in Khartoum, the capital of Sudan, hunting down smallpox cases. From there, he went on to India and Bangladesh.

By the time Francis's obligations to the smallpox campaign were fulfilled, nearly three years had elapsed since he had answered that phone call one morning in Oregon.

Another young American physician, David Heymann, saw a one-shot CDC assignment turn into two years of Indian smallpox-hunting in Bihar and Calcutta. When Heymann's group vaccinated somebody, they always showed pictures of smallpox-stricken Indians and asked for names of people suffering from the disease. In some areas they offered rewards to people who could steer the team to active smallpox cases. If they found a case, the ailing person was quarantined and everybody in the region vaccinated—some against their will.

End Justifies Means

Despite the coercive nature of their activities, few of the fieldworkers doubted that, in the greater scheme of things, what they were doing was just: if 2 million people a year could survive because of momentary inconveniences visited upon a few, then how could there be any doubt about the righteousness of their campaign?

The one concern that did constantly haunt Henderson and his team was the cost of failure. In those brief moments when they allowed themselves to entertain the notion that smallpox might not be eradicated, the scientists knew the world might never again be willing to mobilize across political, national, cultural, racial and religious boundaries to share a common battle against disease. The stakes, clearly, were high.

By the summer of 1974, the WHO team was about to declare victory in Bangladesh, the last stubborn holdout of the virulent variola-major form of smallpox. Officials had even gone so far as to publicly predict that complete elimination of the virus would occur before that November.

But then the rains came, and came, and came. By August, Bangladesh was besieged by water, as dikes and dams burst under the monsoon's force. Refugees poured by the tens of thousands into Dhaka, the nation's capital. Famine spread throughout the land, and the country seemed to be coming apart at the seams. Shortly before the floods, the prime minister, Sheik Mujibur Rahman, was assassinated, and a series of riots, civil violence and coups followed, lasting well into 1975.

After being so close to victory, the task of eliminating—indeed, amid the chaos, *finding*—the remaining cases seemed so daunting that most of the eradication staff gave up. They were exhausted, burnt out.

But French physician Daniel Tarantola told his staff, "Look, this just means we have to get down to micromanagement.... Take it day by day."

Slowly staff confidence and morale were rebuilt, smallpox cases were found, and the enthusiasm returned. Within a year, victory once again seemed within grasp. Heymann and Francis were reporting total success in India, and no new outbreaks had occurred in Africa in months. With all eyes on Bangladesh, excitement rose.

One of the last infected villages was outside the city of Chittagong, which was under the command of an army general. Not knowing what side of the civil war that general was on, or how he felt about foreigners, Tarantola confronted the general and requested permission to vaccinate the villagers. Permission was initially denied, and the disease spread. Once again, it seemed the gigantic obstacles of Bangladesh would force the WHO team to snatch defeat from the jaws of victory.

But the general finally relented, the last outbreak was stifled, and champagne was poured in Dhaka. Tarantola greedily guzzled the champagne, exultant after years of round-the-clock viral pursuit.

The next morning victory once again disappeared when word came that smallpox had surfaced on Bhola, an island off Bangladesh. For the third time the team was forced to remobilize after having been convinced the war was over. This time, when all the affected islanders had been vaccinated, Henderson held his breath a bit before announcing success.

In November 1975, Henderson was able to announce to the world that a three-year-old Bangladesh girl named Rahima Banu had been cured and represented the last case of wild variola major in human history. Two years later, on October 26, 1977, the last case of the less virulent variola minor would be found in Merka, Somalia.

By then Dr. Isao Arita had been in charge of the international effort for 10 months, Henderson having retired. The Japanese physician ran the program with at least as much energy as the tall, bombastic American, but with a personal style that was more low-key and witty.

His humor was put to the test in the Horn of Africa in early 1977, just weeks after military leader Mengistu Haile Mariam seized power in Ethiopia, installing a Soviet-backed, Communist government. The military government in Somalia laid claim to Ogaden, a region then part of eastern Ethiopia, and full-scale war was under way. It was in that area—Ogaden—that the world's last known cases of smallpox variola minor could be found, primarily among Somali Muslims.

Arita knew that UN flags and WHO credentials would offer little protection to his scientific team members in such a volatile situation, yet he also felt time was running out. It was February 1977, and the Hajj was just 10 months away. During the

Hajj, thousands of devout Somali Muslims would make their pilgrimage to Mecca, Saudi Arabia, where they would eat, sleep and pray for several days with some 2 million other followers of Islam from all over the world. If infected pilgrims were part of the Hajj, all efforts to eradicate smallpox would end in failure.

For months the multinational team struggled against the elements, avoided the war's front, and tracked down smallpox cases among the refugees and villagers of Ogaden.

Finally, in Merka, the team found the world's last case of variola minor.

Ali Maow Maalin would be cured, and all forms of smallpox disappeared. Smallpox had been conquered.

Their jobs completed, smallpox team members dispersed to public-health jobs all over the world. Surprisingly, they were not eagerly snatched up by WHO, or congratulated individually for their magnificent efforts. On the contrary, the brash young smallpox scientists were considered arrogant and thoughtless. They violated too many WHO bureaucratic guidelines. And they operated with a single goal in mind—a perspective quite unlike that of those who usually drove the vaguely pro-health WHO and national ministries of health worldwide.

"Science really suffers from bureaucracy," Arita would later declare, adding, "If we hadn't broken every single WHO rule many times over, we would never have defeated smallpox. Never."

Eradication took 11 years, involving about 100 highly trained professionals and thousands of local health workers and staff worldwide. It was achieved at a cost of $300 million.

War on Malaria

A very different outcome awaited those who fought to eradicate malaria worldwide. Between 1958 and 1963 alone, $430 million was spent on a series of failed attempts to eliminate malaria. In 1991 dollars that constituted an expenditure of over $1.9 billion. Between 1964 and 1981, the United States spent an additional $793 million.

When the international effort began, there were millions of

cases of malaria every year, largely concentrated in Southeast Asia and Africa. Though reliable numbers were not available for most parts of the world, it was estimated that, for example, about 1 million people had malaria that year in Sri Lanka, some 100 million in India, and untold numbers, roughly estimated in the "hundreds of millions," in Africa.

On the other hand, humanity possessed powerful weapons. Chloroquine and quinine were effective treatments that, when properly and speedily used, stopped most cases of the disease in a matter of days. And chlorinated-hydrocarbon insecticides—notably DDT—could kill not only adult mosquitoes that carried malarial parasites but their progeny as well, because the chemicals were virtually nonbiodegradable and their insect toxicity could be expected to eliminate pests that landed on sprayed surfaces for months, even years, after chemical treatment.

During the construction of the Panama Canal (1904–14), General William C. Gorgas directed the U.S. Army Medical Corps on a successful campaign to drain swamps, treat local people with quinine, and kill mosquito larvae floating atop pools of water. He did not have DDT at his disposal in those early years, yet the result was virtual eradication of Panamanian malaria. Similar drainage efforts throughout the U.S. Sunbelt were already bringing malaria down to negligible levels by 1947.

Then Egypt embarked on the first successful campaign using DDT to eliminate the *Anopheles gambiae* mosquito. Its initial results were so dramatic that the U.S. Congress allocated $7 million in 1947 for a DDT-based program to eradicate malaria within the 48 states. Five years later, the program was abandoned when not one case of malaria could be found within the U.S. borders.

Similar successes were reported across the European Continent, though malaria stubbornly hung on in parts of Italy, Spain and Greece well into the 1950s. Buoyed by Brazil's success a decade earlier controlling the *A. gambiae* mosquito population, the 1954 Pan American Sanitary Conference held in Santiago,

Chile, resolved to eradicate malaria-carrying mosquitoes from all countries in the Americas, from the Arctic to Antarctica.

In 1956, malariologist Paul Russell, then at Harvard University's School of Public Health, authored a report for the International Development Advisory Board (IDAB) recommending immediate global eradication of malaria. In the report Russell reflected the mainstream scientific views of the day when he argued that DDT was such a powerful tool that a multimillion-dollar worldwide campaign could eliminate all malaria-carrying mosquitoes on the planet within less than a decade.

> Eradication can be pushed through in a community in a period of eight to ten years, with not more than four to six years of actual spraying, without much danger of resistance. But if countries, due to lack of funds, have to proceed slowly, resistance is almost certain to appear and eradication will become economically impossible. *Time is of the essence* [his emphasis] because DDT resistance has appeared in six or seven years.... This is a completely unique moment in the history of man's attack on one of his oldest and most powerful disease enemies. Failure to proceed energetically might postpone malaria eradication indefinitely.

Russell's plan caught the imagination of several key figures in the American political arena of the late 1950s: Secretary of State George Marshall, Senators John F. Kennedy (D-Mass.) and Hubert H. Humphrey (D-Minn.) and President Dwight D. Eisenhower. Though malaria no longer existed in the United States, America was, in 1957, the center of virtually all cash reserves on earth. Europe, Japan and the U.S.S.R. were still smarting from World War II devastation, and what is now called the developing world was largely in the yoke of colonialism or severe underdevelopment. Having won World War II, Americans were of a mind to "fix things up."

Thus, in 1958 Russell's battle for malaria eradication began, backed directly by $23.3 million a year from Congress. Because Russell had been so adamant about the time frame, Congress stipulated that the funds would stop flowing in 1963. In addition to the $23.3 million to be spent annually by IDAB, Congress shelled out funds generously between 1958 and 1963 for WHO (contributing 31 percent of its overall budget and more than 95 percent of its malaria budget), the Pan American Health Organization (PAHO, which got 66 percent of its funds directly from the U.S. Congress), and Unicef (underwriting 40 percent of the UN Children's Fund budget). It was a staggering economic commitment, the equivalent of billions of dollars in 1990. Remarkably, American politicians didn't complain about spending so much money to control diseases few U.S. citizens ever contracted, and the effort enjoyed bipartisan support. President Eisenhower called for the "unconditional surrender" of the microbes, Marshall foresaw the "imminent conquest of disease," and Senator Kennedy predicted that children born in the next decade would no longer face the ancient scourges of pestilence.

The stage was set. The scientists had everything going for them: political support, money, DDT and chloroquine. So certain were they of victory that malaria research came to a virtual halt. Why research something that will no longer exist?

While Congress reviewed Russell's IDAB proposal, Andy Spielman, a young Colorado scientist, took some courses at the Woods Hole Oceanographic Institute in Massachusetts. There he met a middle-aged marine biologist who was quietly rethinking the whole DDT question. She told Spielman that evolution would come between DDT and the dream of malaria eradication. DDT-resistant strains of *Anopheles* mosquitoes were turning up all over the world, she said.

Her name was Rachel Carson, and the same year the United States and WHO embarked on their ambitious campaign to eliminate malarial mosquitoes, Carson started writing *Silent Spring*. Carson never completely opposed pesticide use; rather, she favored their rational and limited application. Prophetically, she worried that widespread agricultural use of insecticides would endanger efforts to control malaria, typhus, African sleeping sickness, yellow fever and encephalitis. She wrote:

The world has heard much of the triumphant war against disease through the control of insect vectors of infection, but it has heard little of the other side of the story—the defeats, the short-lived triumphs that now strongly support the alarming view that the insect enemy has been made stronger by our efforts. Even worse, we may have destroyed our very means of fighting.

She noted that the first public-health use of DDT occurred in 1943. Allied troops sprayed the chemical liberally to eliminate typhus-carrying lice in Italy. The lice were, in fact, killed, and typhus halted, but a year later DDT-resistant *Culex* mosquitoes and houseflies stepped into the vacuum. By 1951, mosquitoes and flies in the region were resistant to DDT, methoxychlor, chlordane, heptachlor and benzene hexachloride, and Italians had returned to time-honored tactics for insect control: screened windows, flypaper and flyswatters.

In 1959 Spielman joined the faculty of the Harvard School of Public Health and discovered that no courses on malaria or *Anopheles* mosquitoes were on the curriculum. With the leader of the world's malaria-eradication campaign on the faculty, it was considered distasteful to offer such courses. Training young scientists in techniques of mosquito control implied that Russell's efforts would fail and such knowledge would actually be necessary for future practitioners of public health.

Malaria had, indeed, reached its nadir. But it had not been eliminated. In some countries success was so close that people were already celebrating. Sri Lanka, for example, had 1 million malaria cases in 1955; just 18 in 1963.

But a deal's a deal. Russell promised success by 1963, and Congress was in no mood to entertain extending funds for another year, or two. As far as Congress was concerned, failure to reach eradication by 1963 simply meant it couldn't be done, in any time frame. And at the time virtually all the spare cash was American; without steady infusions of U.S. dollars, the effort died abruptly.

In 1963 Harvard put malaria control back on its curriculum.

As malaria relentlessly increased again after 1963, developing countries were forced to commit ever-larger amounts of scarce public-health dollars to the problem. India, for example, dedicated over a third of its entire health budget in 1965 to malaria control.

Everything started to unravel. The Green Revolution—a World Bank-backed scheme to improve Third World economies through large-scale cash-crop production—got under way. Turning thousands of acres of formerly diversely planted and fallow land into monocultured farms for export production of coffee, rice, sorghum, wheat, pineapples, or other cash crops necessitated ever-increasing pesticide use. When an area had very diverse plant life, its insect population was also diverse and no single pest species generally had an opportunity to so dominate that it could destroy a crop. As plant diversity decreased, however, competition and predation among insects also declined. As a result, croplands could be overwhelmed rapidly by destructive insects. Farmers responded during the 1960s with heavy pesticide use, which often worked in the short term. But in the long run, pesticides usually killed off beneficial insects, while the crop-attacking pests became resistant to chemicals. A vicious cycle set in, forcing use of a wider assortment of insecticides to protect crops.

At the very time malaria-control efforts were splintering or collapsing, the agricultural use of DDT and its sister compounds was soaring. Almost overnight resistant mosquito populations appeared all over the world.

As Russell kept a worried eye on the pesticide-resistance problem, a new crisis appeared: two people who were taking chloroquine developed malaria in South America. Almost simultaneously, chloroquine-resistant malaria turned up in Colombia, Thailand, Venezuela and Brazil. The drug had been in use for only 15 years; widespread use spanned less than a decade's time. By 1950 a second drug, primaquine, was available and many countries returned to the use of the ancient antimalarial, quinine. But resistance soon developed to those and other drugs introduced in the 1960s. By 1963 U.S. forces fighting in Vietnam encountered chloroquine-resistant malaria, and the Army began a major effort to research and develop new antimalarial drugs.

The drug-resistant problem could only have been aggravated by government decisions in some countries—notably Papua New Guinea—to add chloroquine to all table salt.

By the time the smallpox campaign was approaching victory in 1975, parasite resistance to chloroquine and mosquito resistance to DDT and other pesticides were both so widespread that nobody spoke of eliminating malaria. Increasingly, experts saw the grand smallpox success as an aberration, rather than a goal that could easily be replicated with other diseases.

In 1975 the worldwide incidence of malaria was about 2.5 times what it had been in 1961, midway through Russell's campaign. In some countries the disease was claiming horrendous numbers of people. China, for example, had an estimated 9 million cases in 1975, compared to about 1 million in 1961. India jumped in that time period from 1 million to over 6 million cases.

A new global iatrogenic form of malaria was emerging— "iatrogenic" meaning created as a result of medical treatment. In its well-meaning zeal to treat the world's malaria scourge, humanity had created a new epidemic.

2

Global Program on AIDS

J ONATHAN MANN was tremendously excited. True, there were any number of things that could still go awry; diplomatic noses might start bleeding, political shenanigans could well break out. But he and his highly energetic—and sly—staff of WHO's Global Program on AIDS (GPA) had for months carefully and strategically planned for this day.

"We are entering a new era," Mann had assured an international press corps. "We will make 1988 the year we turn the tide against the AIDS [acquired immunodeficiency syndrome] virus."

He looked out over the largest gathering of ministers of health ever assembled. Of the representatives of 148 nations who now sat before him in the vast Queen Elizabeth II Conference Center in London, 117 were ministers of health or their country's equivalent. Every key nation, save one, was represented by the most politically powerful health official in their land: Mann was ashamed to say that the exception was his own country. Still not wishing to give AIDS a priority status, the

Reagan Administration sent Dr. Robert Windom, who ranked two notches down the power ladder from the secretary of health and human services, Otis Bowen.

Never in history had the majority of the world's top health officials gathered to discuss an epidemic. No scourge—not malaria, smallpox, yellow fever, or the plague—had ever commanded such diplomatic attention. Some 700 delegates and 400 journalists were also present in the London hall on this ice-cold January morning in 1988 to witness the World Summit of Ministers of Health on Programs for AIDS Prevention. Mann felt that it was a coup for his program, for WHO, and for millions of powerless people with AIDS.

Mann urgently hoped to drive home a message to the world's health leadership: AIDS is spreading; if it hasn't yet emerged in your country, it will, unless you plan now, follow our recommendations, educate your populations, and embrace condom-based programs as a prevention strategy.

As of January 26, 1988, 75,392 cases of AIDS had officially been reported to WHO. But that figure was a gross understatement of the true dimensions of the pandemic: most nations lacked genuine systems for amassing and recording such health statistics. Mann tactfully didn't mention from the podium what everyone in the audience knew to be true; namely, that many nations were deliberately covering up their epidemics for political and economic reasons. Such delicate issues would be dealt with later, in private arm-twistings and minister-to-minister preplanned strategic confrontations.

Mann differentiated the ways in which the AIDS virus was spreading from person to person. In what he called Pattern I countries, such as those of North America and Western Europe, AIDS was spreading primarily via the sharing of needles between intravenous drug users and sexually among gay men. In Pattern II countries, such as those of Africa, AIDS was a heterosexual disease.

Though he was cautious in his public choice of words, it was Pattern III nations that most concerned Mann as he spoke in London. Asia, the Communist bloc, the largely Muslim Middle

East, and much of the Pacific region had only very tiny out-breaks of AIDS.

Pattern III, in other words, represented the political future of the worldwide AIDS epidemic. There was still a window of opportunity for public-health action that might successfully prevent HIV (human immunodeficiency virus) from emerging in the majority of the world's populations.

Many of the Pattern III political leaders had already recognized the threat of HIV importation, of course, and taken their own steps to curb such events. However, Mann and his staff, which included smallpox hero Tarantola, were appalled by many of the antiemergence measures some countries had taken. Privately, Tarantola had already spent months flying all over the world in attempts to convince many of the same ministers who now sat in the London conference hall that AIDS wasn't anything like smallpox. There was no vaccine that one could require that immigrants and visitors receive. The virus didn't manifest itself symptomatically for years—perhaps over a decade—in ways that indicated its presence even to the infected individual. And the AIDS blood test wasn't foolproof.

"What are you going to do, test every immigrant five or six times a year, every visiting student once a week? If you think you can keep the virus out of your country with legislation and testing, you are wrong," Tarantola told public-health officials.

London Summit Crucial to AIDS Control

Mann was worried that the world would become a patchwork of repressive public-health regimes with laws aimed at keeping a virus, as well as its potential carriers—gays, Africans, prostitutes, drug users, poor immigrants—out. He feared that it would push populations that already existed at the margins of global society further away from the mainstream, from medicine and all hopes of disease control. Indeed, restrictions intended to control populations at greatest danger for HIV infection might actually have the reverse effect, exacerbating the social and economic conditions in their lives that drove them to adopt risky behaviors. Simply put, he felt certain that his mo-

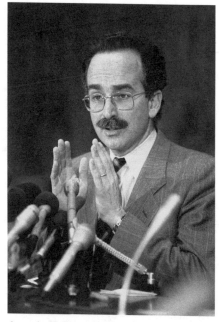

Dr. Jonathan Mann, epidemiologist, who headed seminal AIDS research project in Zaire before becoming director of WHO's Global Program on AIDS in Geneva, Switzerland (1986–90).

UPI/Corbis-Bettmann

ment in London was pivotal to deciding whether HIV's emergence in most countries would be prevented through education of local populaces or temporarily stalled by repressive laws.

As a scientist, Mann knew that the men and women now looking up at him on the dais, studying his smile and careful public modesty, were "people of politics." What the ministers said publicly here in London would be at least as much for domestic consumption as for the sake of any global effort to stop the pandemic.

Anticipating such limitations, Mann and his GPA staff had toiled for months in preparation for this moment. Lifelong WHO veterans, and occasional renegades, Tarantola and Manuel Carballo, showed Mann how to maneuver around the labyrinthine and often byzantine UN bureaucracy. Swiss-American Tom Netter, having spent years covering the rise of the Solidarity labor movement and the fall of communism in Poland for the Associated Press, plotted every step of GPA's interactions with the international media. Spanish-born Carballo, who knew every nook and cranny of WHO even better than WHO Director General Halfdan Mahler, helped spot the few potentially influential individuals within the bureaucracy who understood the urgency of the AIDS epidemic.

"This is a place where people put URGENT! on requests for pencil supplies," Mann said in wonder. "The concept of genuinely dire emergency has almost no meaning here."

When Mann had originally left Kinshasa, capital of Zaire, to take the reins of power in Geneva in November 1986, he had a total working budget of $5 million, a part-time secretary, and three epidemiologists who were borrowed from other programs. Mann's own salary was still paid by CDC.

By the time he reached London for the January 1988 summit, less than two years later, 40-year-old Mann commanded a far-flung AIDS program, a considerable staff, and a budget of over $50 million, with $92 million promised for 1989. It was, by WHO bureaucratic standards, a meteoric rise.

While Mann, Tarantola, Heymann, Carballo and the rest of the AIDS staff did their best to create a highly publicized sense of worldwide emergency and mobilization, jealousy simmered in the hallways of the vast Geneva complex. In the enormous vaulted lobby of WHO headquarters, experts on cholera, malaria, diarrheal diseases, schistosomiasis, health economics, polio and vaccine development gathered in discrete clusters by the three-story-high glass wall that afforded a view of Lake Geneva and Mont Blanc. And they whispered. They cited the GPA's own statistics on AIDS—those modest numbers of underreported cases—and asked why the new disease should command such resources and attention when other microbes were killing tens of millions of people. They noted that Mann and some other GPA staffers were Americans, and assured one another that all the concern was *only* in place because AIDS was killing homosexuals in New York and San Francisco.

Mann and his team either were oblivious to the talk behind their backs or chose to ignore it. In either case, when questioned directly about comparisons between WHO commitments to, for example, malaria versus AIDS, the GPA group would say that all global health programs were underfunded and not one dollar or yen of AIDS monies should be gathered at the expense of other health efforts.

And they would politely remind critics that AIDS was a newly emerging epidemic which, by definition, would swell to claim tens of millions of lives if not stopped immediately. On that point Mann enjoyed the full support of the director-general.

The staff of GPA discussed quite consciously among themselves the inherent contradictions in the need for a state of emergency to halt a newly emerging disease versus the essential nature of WHO and the UN system. Though outbreaks of Ebola, Marburg and Lassa and other emergencies had received the quick attention of WHO, they couldn't serve as models for action against AIDS. First of all, each had surfaced as seemingly confined local emergencies. Second, they, at least in part, burned out on their own. Third, the microbes caused almost immediate disease in those who were infected, with an alarming level of mortality; there could be no doubt to the populaces or their governments that a state of emergency was warranted. Fourth, fairly simple measures, such as provision of sterile syringes, could stop the primary spread of the diseases.

AIDS Slow to Trigger Alarm

In contrast, HIV surfaced almost simultaneously on three continents and was quickly a feature on the health horizons of at least 20 different nations. Not only was there no sign that AIDS might burn out on its own; scientists could see no evidence of the famous bell-shaped curve of infection and disease. Far from causing immediate disease and death, HIV was a slow burner that hid deep inside people's lymph nodes, often for over a decade, before producing detectable infections. As a result, a society could already have thousands of infected citizens before any sound of alarm was rung, and even when the first AIDS cases appeared, their numbers were small enough to allow governments to feel comfortable about ignoring the seemingly trifling problem. Denial was all too easy a response to AIDS.

Furthermore, no facile measures could be taken by a government to bring AIDS to a halt. Unlike Ebola, Marburg, drug-resistant cerebral malaria, or Lassa, HIV hit specific social targets. It was a sexual disease. It was associated with homosexuality, promiscuity and drug abuse. It pitted public health against organized religion and the moral pillars of society.

It was, in short, easy to ignore and uncomfortable to confront.

WHO, acutely aware of the unsettling aspects of AIDS, initially chose the first route—ignoring the emerging disease. From 1981 to late 1986 barely a whisper about AIDS emanated from Geneva. By the time Mann and his crew started sounding every alarm they could get their hands on, HIV had successfully emerged and reached full-fledged epidemic status in all the major cities of North America and Western Europe, as well as most of the urban centers of sub-Saharan Africa.

Rubbing against the bureaucratic grain, the GPA staff group moved with both haste and deliberation. They decided on a strategy for control of AIDS in which vaccine and drug-research efforts, already under way in key wealthy nations, received the GPA's encouragement but not significant emphasis. With no cure in sight, the GPA's best focus, they felt, was on prevention of further spread of HIV. Though details would come much later, during 1987 the GPA outlined the need for national AIDS programs in every country—programs that would coordinate mass education campaigns about the disease. Societal awareness was the first step—that was Tarantola's job. To prevent further spread of HIV it was crucial that every nation's blood banks be free of HIV, sterile syringes had to be available to health providers, and people who were infected with HIV had to be counseled carefully so that they couldn't pass their virus on to others. Counseling was Carballo's job. Anti-AIDS programs had to be coordinated not only within countries but worldwide.

And perhaps most important in Mann's mind was the need to eliminate the atmosphere of discrimination and prejudice that surrounded every aspect of AIDS.

"Discrimination simply drives AIDS underground," Mann

repeatedly asserted. "The epidemic doesn't go away, it simply becomes harder to see, more alienated from public health. If you drive it underground, you guarantee its spread."

First UN Resolution on a Specific Disease

With those vague principles in mind, the GPA targeted sequentially each of the international bodies whose support the GPA staff felt was crucial. On May 15, 1987, the 40th World Health Assembly, the legislative body of WHO, passed the Global Strategy for the Prevention and Control of AIDS, endorsing the strategy of the Global Program on AIDS. That gave the GPA its mandate, power and seal of approval. And on October 26, 1987, Mann did something no WHO functionary at his level had ever done: he addressed the General Assembly of the UN. For the first time in its history the UN passed a resolution on a specific disease, formally endorsing WHO's leadership in the war against AIDS.

Over the next three months, the GPA staff carefully prepared for the London summit, further detailing its strategy for control of the emerging pandemic, collecting data on the epidemic's scope, and carefully monitoring the AIDS-related activities of governments around the world. Though they loudly decried all attempts to keep AIDS at bay through legislation against HIV-positive individuals or members of social groups considered at greatest risk for exposure to the virus, the GPA members watched helplessly as 81 nations passed such laws. As the new year and the London summit approached, at least 10 more governments were debating passage of similar legislation and the international mood was growing ugly.

In the Middle East, tough laws in some Islamic countries passed in 1986–87 made failure to submit to HIV tests and "promiscuous" behavior punishable by imprisonment.

In Western Europe, the European Economic Community repeatedly condemned all efforts to legislatively restrict the travels, employment, or reasonable freedoms of people infected with HIV. Nevertheless, laws and condemnations were forthcoming. Belgium, West Germany, Greece, Finland and Spain all passed new legislation, or interpreted preexisting public-health law, to permit expulsion or visa denial to HIV-positive foreigners who were seeking work permits or student credentials. In practice, these regulations were primarily directed against Africans and, in the case of Germany, Turks.

The Eastern bloc and the Soviet Union posed special difficulties for Mann and his colleagues, because, in general, the Communist states claimed not to have much—or any—AIDS, and they wanted to keep it that way.

The Soviet Union, after long denying that it had any indigenous AIDS cases, issued fiats in late 1987 requiring testing of most foreigners and giving the KGB (state security) and the police powers to order HIV tests—refusal punishable by imprisonment—on its citizens.

Elsewhere in the Communist world two nations clearly stood out: Cuba and China.

No nation on earth had ordered as broad a sweep of AIDS regulations as had Cuba. Between March 1986 and January 1988 the government conducted 1,534,993 HIV tests, according to the Ministry of Health, and the intention was to test every citizen and nontourist visitor to the country, or 10.4 million people.

By January 1988 the Cuban government had identified 174 HIV-positive individuals and placed them under lifetime quarantine. Several of the infected people were recently returned veterans of the Angolan civil war, in which Cuban military advisers played a pivotal role in defense of the Luanda (Angolan) government. More than 300,000 Cubans returned from Angola between 1975 and 1987; HIV-1 was clearly present and causing AIDS in Angola at least as early as 1983.

In the People's Republic of China there were also practices under way that troubled the GPA. Beginning in December 1986, the Chinese government instituted mandatory testing for all foreign students; in reality, the edict was carried out with greatest vigor on Americans and Africans. Students who failed to comply with the tests were barred entry or deported. The mandatory testing list had expanded by 1987 to include all foreigners who wished to stay in China for more than a year and all Chinese citizens returning from overseas.

By the time the world's health ministers gathered in London for their AIDS summit, China had already tested more than 10,000 foreign students, 20,000 returning Chinese students, and thousands of foreign businessmen: all in a period of less than four months. In addition, the Chinese government issued strict laws against "illicit sexual contact with foreigners," which included all forms of nonmarital sex. All foreigners caught having such relations with Chinese citizens could be deported, and the government stipulated that entertaining local citizens in one's hotel room—regardless of what actually transpired in the room—would be considered in violation of the law.

Asia Represents Special Threat

Asia was a very special concern for WHO; though AIDS hadn't yet emerged in most of the area, those familiar with social and medical practices in much of the region felt sure that the virus could easily overwhelm the continent. WHO Director General Mahler predicted that a "major catastrophe" loomed for Asia if the continent failed to come to grips with AIDS and specifically named India, Bangladesh, Thailand, Indonesia and the Philippines as countries at greatest risk.

Thailand had a thriving sex and prostitution trade. Long a major source of foreign exchange for the nation, the prostitution and "entertainment services" industry swelled radically during the Vietnam War, as Thailand was designated an official R and R (rest and recreation) site for U.S. military personnel. By the end of the war Thailand's revenues from the sex trade equaled a quarter of all rice-trade income. Not wishing to call attention to potential problems in so lucrative an industry, the Thai government ignored all WHO pleas to institute nationwide AIDS-education campaigns and promote condom use. Instead, Thailand alternately tried to repress or ignore the virus, imprisoning some HIV-positive foreigners while issuing so-called AIDS-free certificates to male and female prostitutes who serviced tourists.

India also perceived AIDS as a foreign problem and declined to conduct any form of domestic AIDS education. By the end of 1986 India had in place laws requiring HIV tests of all foreign students. As was the case in so many other countries, these laws were almost exclusively—and often brutally—enforced against African students.

Despite such measures, by mid-1987 scattered surveys of female prostitutes in India were already revealing that AIDS was emerging in the country. As the numbers of documented AIDS cases in India rose during 1987, the Ministry of Health declared that foreign students and tourists were chiefly responsible, as were "foreign priests attending Christian conventions."

Other Asian countries responded with similar antiforeigner laws and actions, notably Japan, South Korea, Indonesia, Malaysia and Singapore.

The GPA staff scrambled to convince Asian leaders that such policies would only hinder efforts to prevent the emergence of an enormous AIDS epidemic on the continent. But the Asian nations correctly pointed out that their policies were modeled after those of the most powerful nation on earth, the home of Jonathan Mann, the country leading the world's AIDS research effort, the nation with the greatest number of officially reported AIDS cases: namely, the United States of America.

Deep Divisions over AIDS Policy

The Reagan Administration's (1981–89) decision to follow an overall policy of trying to control AIDS through the use of legal instruments was a huge thorn in Mann's side. At a time when the GPA was stressing public education as the primary tool for preventing the spread of HIV, the U.S. government was torn asunder by sentiments that *no* form of tax-funded AIDS education should be permitted. And tensions at the White House mirrored a severely dichotomous response toward the AIDS epidemic at the level of grass-roots America. All across the country by 1986 the populace was deeply divided between those who favored a nonjudgmental education-driven approach to the epidemic and those who wanted HIV-positive people and members of identified high-risk groups segregated by some means from the rest of society.

The foci of attack were homosexuals, "immoral lifestyles," drug users and sinners—the purported purveyors of viral ruin. Like their Islamic counterparts in the Middle East, many Christian political leaders in the United States were convinced that there was a religious message to be derived from AIDS, an epidemic that would best be stopped through moral virtue.

In his first major speech addressing the AIDS epidemic, delivered before the College of Physicians in Philadelphia, Pennsylvania, on April 2, 1987, President Ronald Reagan assured the nation—for the first time—that he was concerned about AIDS and considered it "Public Enemy Number One."

"The federal role must be to give educators accurate information about the disease. How that information is used must be up to schools and parents, not government," Reagan said. "But let's be honest with ourselves. AIDS information cannot be what some call 'value neutral.' After all, when it comes to preventing AIDS, don't medicine and morality teach the same lessons?...I think that abstinence has been lacking in much of the education."

The President's comments reflected an ongoing dispute within his Administration over the proper tactics for control of AIDS and prevention of the emergence of HIV in geographic and demographic parts of the country not yet touched by the virus. Reagan's surgeon-general, Dr. C. Everett Koop, wanted frank discussion of abstention, the AIDS epidemic and safe sex to be conducted in the nation's schools. But Reagan's secretary of education, William Bennett, adamantly opposed such plans, favoring instead efforts to identify and control HIV carriers through compulsory HIV testing of all hospital patients, marriage license applicants, prison inmates and foreigners applying for immigration visas.

Vice President George Bush was straddling his roles as adviser to Reagan and candidate for the presidency. He played to voters on the right, calling for mandatory marriage license HIV tests and public identification of people who were infected.

It all came to a head in Washington, D.C., June 1–5, 1987.

More than 10,000 scientists, physicians and reporters descended upon the nation's capital for the Third International Conference on AIDS.

The keynote speaker, U.S. Surgeon General Koop, dressed in his starched white Public Health Service uniform, looked at the sea of enthusiastic scientists and activists with genuine surprise. What began as a polite reception swelled into nearly hysterical cheering, chanting, shouting and foot-stomping as thousands of activists and American scientists signaled their support for Koop's dissident position within the Reagan Administration. Koop was stunned. Just two years earlier most of the people in the room would have booed him off the stage because of his staunch, often radical opposition to abortion. But now they gave him a hero's welcome unlike any the 71-year-old Brooklyn-born physician had experienced.

In contrast, when presidential candidate Bush took to the podium, activists stood silently, their backs turned to the Vice President, many holding placards aloft condemning Reagan Administration policies. Cameras rolled, photographers' bulbs flashed, and hundreds of scientists stood one by one to join the activists in turning their backs on the Vice President of the United States.

"AIDS is a touchstone of politics, of racism, of bigotry," Mann told the conferees. "We see a rising wave of stigmatism around the world. AIDS has become a threat to free travel and global movement. People all over the world are seeking answers— simple answers—as the pandemic spreads. People are promoting sex cards, tattoos, quarantines, police lists, deportations, home burnings, incarcerations of select population groups.

"How our societies treat HIV-positive individuals will test our collective moral strength. This test will present itself with increasing challenge in the coming years."

Though Mann's remarks received thunderous applause that day in Washington and were carried by the media worldwide, the message many powerful politicians derived from the Third International Conference on AIDS was quite the opposite. They saw shouting homosexuals showing disrespect for national leaders and upstart scientists daring to tell them how to govern. And they didn't like it.

Two weeks after the close of the AIDS conference the U.S. Senate voted unanimously—96 to 0—to mandate HIV tests for all applicants for legal immigration to the United States. That same week, governors of three states—Minnesota, Texas and Colorado—signed laws permitting local authorities to quarantine indefinitely HIV-positive individuals who seemed by virtue of their sexual activities to pose a threat to society.

By the time the world's ministers of health gathered two months later in London, the United States had federal laws requiring HIV tests of foreign students, immigrants, longtime visitors, all military personnel and applicants for military service, U.S. overseas foreign-service personnel and applicants for the domestic youth employment service called the Job Corps. Entry to the United States could be barred to any noncitizen known to be HIV-positive, and though Bush had in oratory opposed discrimination against people with AIDS, HIV-positive applicants for foreign-service, military, or Job Corps positions were, by law, denied employment.

AIDS: A Multifaceted Epidemic

Before the London meeting, the GPA staff had reviewed all the legal and political activities surrounding AIDS and concluded that they were witnessing, in slow motion, many of the same social responses that had followed the arrival of the plague in fourteenth-century Europe. In both cases there were actually three different social epidemics within the larger biological epidemic.

First, with the initial emergence of the microbe—plague bacteria or HIV—came denial in all tiers of society. The tendency was to ignore the microbial threat, or assume only "they"—some distinct subpopulation of society—were at risk. The microbes exploited such denial, spreading rapidly while humans made no attempts, through their personal or collective behaviors, to block any of the avenues of transmission of the organisms.

The second social epidemic was fear. Some event in the

biological epidemic would suddenly shock a society out of its state of denial, propelling people into a state of group terror. In fourteenth-century Europe, it was often the plague death of a popular cleric or a local lord or the sudden public expiration of a child that prompted panic. The timescale was quick: plague-infested rats might arrive in a town on Tuesday, local human deaths might begin in the harbor area by Thursday or Friday, and a riveting event could spark widespread panic by the middle of the following week.

But AIDS was a slow killer, and the biological epidemic unfolded in each country over a span of many months or years. So the first social-denial stage might persist for over a decade. Fear might also linger for years, giving rise to all sorts of panic responses and inappropriate actions, such as setting fire to the home of two HIV-positive children with hemophilia in Florida.

Eventually, the GPA staff knew, the social epidemic of fear usually yielded to a wake of repression. Fear-driven government response was usually irrational, prompting attacks on the victims of disease, rather than the microbes. During the plague such fear-driven repression led to the wholesale slaughter of Jews and of women accused of witchcraft. Though outright genocide certainly hadn't surfaced in response to AIDS, Mann's staff felt certain that in the absence of strong political leadership guiding populaces toward rationality, the epidemic could have violent consequences in some societies.

As HIV emerged in new areas of the world, Mann hoped to find a way to break this chain of social epidemics; to push governments out of denial before they had an epidemic on their hands; or failing that, to move a society out of fear to effective action, rather than panic-driven repression. The GPA group knew that they were breaking new ground, that few societies had ever in history responded wisely or rationally to major epidemics, and that lessons learned with AIDS could be applied to combating future emergences of all sorts of microbes. They searched for answers.

At the GPA, Carballo said that the epidemic was forcing researchers all over the world to evaluate—and reevaluate—the effectiveness of a whole battery of standard public-health weapons, in hopes that something besides a chilling death toll could motivate individuals and governments to take rational steps to protect themselves from the virus.

Those at Greatest Risk from AIDS Hardest to Reach

"What makes the AIDS effort especially difficult," Carballo said one afternoon shortly before the London summit, "is that those who are at greatest risk are those who are divorced from traditional values and culture. They have had to innovate new cultures. They find friends in bars and clubs. And nothing in the relationships is stable."

Without social stability, people were hard to reach, whether they were gay men frequenting bars in San Francisco, migrant workers in Mexico, newly urbanized young women in Kinshasa, Zaire, Burmese prostitutes in Bangkok, the Thai capital, or injecting drug users in the Bronx. Such people were deeply separated from the traditional mores of their respective societies, often cut off from their families and mainstream workplaces.

In the 1960s, French-born American bacteriologist René Dubos wrote extensively about the special vulnerability to the microbes among people who lived lives of poverty. History demonstrated repeatedly that, with rare exceptions, the microbes exploited the weak points of economically bereft lives: chronic malnutrition, prostitution, alcoholism, dense housing, poor hygiene and egregious working conditions.

Carballo and his colleagues recognized that there was more to microbial vulnerability than the social-class arguments put forward by Dubos. When information was the key to self-protection, there were gradations of Homo sapiens vulnerability that, yes, could be rooted in economic class, but could also stem from social alienation. People who were treated as outcasts from the dominant culture in which they lived could be denied vital life-protecting information or public-health tools. If the larger society reviled a particular subgroup, its marginalization could be a risk factor, Carballo argued, every bit as crucial as a contaminated syringe.

Carballo saw a confluence of social factors at play in the emergence of HIV in societies: marginalization, social alienation, poverty and discrimination. In his mind, they united to form a social bridge across which HIV traveled into one society after another.

On January 28, 1988, the London summit endorsed the GPA's 15-point declaration that called for openness and candor between governments and scientists, opposed AIDS-related discrimination, gave primacy to national education programs as means to limit the spread of AIDS, and reaffirmed the GPA's role in international leadership. Mann and Mahler viewed it as a triumph.

Summit Declaration Has Limited Success

But even as they smiled for the cameras and signed the declaration, seeds of failure were being sown. The declaration said nothing directly about quarantines, immigration policies, or forced deportations, delegates to the summit having concluded that no agreement on those pivotal issues could be reached between the 149 nations. Worse yet, representatives of critically important countries—like China and the U.S.S.R.—openly scoffed at the GPA's attempts to promote educative efforts over restrictive measures. China's delegate denied the existence of homosexuals, drug users and prostitutes in his country, thus insisting AIDS couldn't threaten the People's Republic. And Soviet Minister of Health Yevgeny Chazov insisted that Slavic genetic superiority had rendered the populace immune to the virus.

Despite the efforts of the GPA, the pandemic spread relentlessly, always emerging first in communities that were on the outer periphery of societies' margins.

With each passing day in 1988, Mann became more strongly convinced that disease emergence was a human-rights issue, in the strictest legal sense of the phrase. Though the physician/scientist had never before been exposed to international human-rights law, some of those working around him had—particularly Katarina Tomasevski, an attorney and public-health expert who served as a consultant to the GPA. Tomasevski introduced Mann to the body of international human-rights law. And Mann, in turn, increasingly framed GPA policy pronouncements on such issues as international freedom to travel, HIV screening of refugees, access to health care for prostitutes, and discrimination against homosexuals in the context of the major instruments of human-rights law. Tomasevski demonstrated that most of the government actions the GPA found repugnant, such as deportation of HIV-positive Africans from Asian countries following enforced testing and detention, were violations of international legal pacts to which the offending nations had previously agreed.

While the staff of the GPA became more outspoken about the connection they perceived between human rights and the spread of HIV, anger and jealousy were building all around them. Some critics began dropping hints to the international press corps about "left-wingers in Geneva." Among Mahler's top aides were men who made no bones about their feelings that the GPA was reflecting "homosexual politics." Human rights, though a topic of serious discussion within most other UN agencies, had never received much attention at WHO.

"Medical people think of human rights as torture and so on. They don't think of it as what they do. And they certainly don't think of a constitutional right to health care," WHO rights expert Sev Fluss explained.

"When AIDS first emerged, our response was disastrous," Fluss conceded. "People thought it was like Ebola and Marburg, which went away without creating a global epidemic. A flash in the pan, that's what they thought."

But as early as 1983, 10 countries passed legislation specifically targeting AIDS, and Fluss thought it rather intriguing that a new disease was prompting so many laws. By the time the GPA was established, 21 more countries had passed major AIDS legislation, and Fluss had an office designated as the WHO Health Legislation Unit. But the HIV pandemic kept spreading, right past all those laws, national border patrols, HIV-testing centers, and alleged human genetic superiority.

Within nations it spread to new population groups, made its way from urban centers to rural areas, crossed class boundaries. Between nations it surmounted virtually every obstacle, save condoms, that humans placed in its way—and certainly each legislative barrier.

3

Africa: AIDS Imperils World's Poorest Nations

By 1988 Western economists and African leaders were asking out loud, "Will this epidemic slow, or even destroy, African development? Is it possible that AIDS will destroy all the development programs we have spent the last three decades building?"

The disease, which so recently had been added to the agenda of international human rights, was also becoming a bona fide macroeconomic issue, threatening both fiscal and social development in the world's poorest nations. It seemed too horrible to contemplate, yet inescapably apparent, that the global AIDS pandemic might well make the world's poorest nations much, much poorer. After years of struggling to rise above Third World status, these nations might be slipping backward on a wave of "Thirdworldization."

The World Bank's Mead Over pioneered much of the research on the economic impact of AIDS in Africa, which between 1988 and 1993 was supplemented greatly by the research of economists, mathematical modelers and epidemiologists in the United States, U.K., France and at WHO.

They began their calculations with several key assumptions: first, that African nations entered the AIDS era already severely impoverished. For example, the 1987 gross national product (GNP) per capita in the United States was $16,690. In Tanzania it was $290, in Zaire a mere $170.

Second, no African nation faced a single epidemic crisis. Since the 1970s a host of new microbes had successfully emerged and swept across the continent: drug-resistant malaria, drug-resistant tuberculosis, urbanized yellow fever, Rift Valley fever and waves of measles epidemics, to name a few. That meant that the health care systems of African nations were already stretched to their limits. Given scarce resources for health care—averaging $1.00 to $10 per capita annually—any additional burden seriously endangered the viability of entire national medical systems.

Compounding the problem was the seeming synergy between microbial epidemics. Wherever AIDS became endemic, tuberculosis followed closely. One epidemic sparked another; malaria and HIV fed upon one another, as did cytomegalovirus, Epstein-Barr virus, syphilis, gonorrhea, chancroid and a host of others. Though no one had a detailed empirical grasp of the relationships, it was clear throughout Africa that wave upon wave of infectious diseases influenced one another and further taxed the health care systems and economies of afflicted nations.

A third assumption was that AIDS would have a uniquely harsh impact because of who in Africa were the microbe's primary targets. Studies all over the continent showed that among the hardest-hit social groups was the well-educated urban elite. These were the young adults who had attended universities in Boston, Oxford, Moscow and Paris, acquiring skills that could be used to navigate their countries out of postcolonial stagnation into prosperity and infrastructural order. But they were also among the few Africans who possessed disposable incomes and could afford to indulge in the carefree nightlife of cities like Kinshasa, Nairobi (Kenya), Harare (Zimbabwe), and Yaoundé

(Cameroon). Long before anyone had heard of AIDS, the continent's educated elite was unknowingly becoming infected in the discos, brothels and nightclubs of Africa's glittering nocturnal ambience. To economists, who placed productivity values on human lives, that meant that AIDS was taking a particularly sharp toll on Africa's future.

A fourth consideration was the familial nature of the epidemic. In Africa, whole families seemed to die off, each survivor's burden increased by the need to care for the sick and compensate for the decline in family income brought about by the deaths of adult providers. In some devastated areas, such as the Lake Victoria region, familial destruction led to the economic collapse of whole villages. And, with time, that could have a ripple effect through all tiers of the regional economy.

All economic forecasts had to begin with estimates of the size

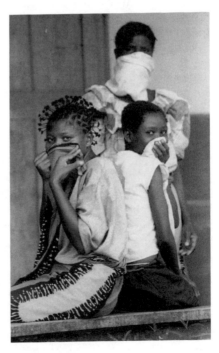

Zairian health workers cover their faces outside isolation ward at Kikwit hospital during Ebola epidemic of 1995, in which more than 250 people died.

Such outbreaks are deadly but do not pose the long-term threat to society that AIDS does.

and forecasted scope of a country's current epidemic. Nobody, however, including those who reported countries' AIDS statistics, believed that the officially reported number came close to reflecting the true scope of the HIV/AIDS epidemics in developing countries. But what was the reality?

Some African countries were still holding back accurate information about the scope of their epidemics as late as 1990, particularly when sensitive groups—such as the military—evidenced high infection rates. Still other countries were overwhelmed by famines, civil wars and political instabilities that rendered the business of disease record-keeping all but impossible. And all African countries were hampered by severe infrastructural problems that hindered diagnosis, treatment and reporting of AIDS.

HIV infection rates in some groups were already staggering by 1988 and would reach positively horrendous proportions by 1993, when some studies would find, for example, that upward of 40 percent of women of reproductive age in key African cities carried the virus.

AIDS' Economic Impact

Even without solid epidemic estimates, economists who were paying attention to Africa's pandemic were, as early as January 1988, predicting financial hard times for the continent: patchworks of small-scale famines; "an economic disaster" based on the direct costs of AIDS care, HIV-testing costs, a year's supply of condoms, AZT (azidothymine) and other drugs for opportunistic infections (where such pharmaceuticals were at all available); and loss of net industrial and agricultural productivity due to deceased work force. They warned that AIDS was creating "a global underclass," over and above the previously existent world community of impoverished individuals.

The real question was whether the AIDS epidemic might destroy the Third World's arduous efforts to pull itself out of perpetual poverty and disease into political stability and economic growth. After the expenditures of billions of dollars of foreign aid and loans from wealthy nations—and after accruing massive debts—some of the world's poorest nations were just beginning to turn the tide.

Jonathan Mann felt it essential to get a handle on the development issue, not only because it was intrinsically important but also because solid empirical answers to the economic question would most likely affect investments in AIDS prevention programs at the international, national and local levels.

The task fell to the GPA's Jim Chin. A year earlier Chin had been running infectious diseases programs for the state of California, living a comfortable, albeit generally routine, life in Berkeley. There, he had commanded a staff of about 400 people and oversaw an annual $65 million budget. In 1989, however, the cautious American found himself facing the formidable task of forecasting the fate of a continent. With a total staff of five people and a tiny piece of the GPA's $90 million budget, Chin toiled in a cramped Geneva office.

Chin collaborated with Tanzanian scientist S. K. Lwangwa to develop models that, first, could determine how many unreported AIDS cases were currently occurring in Africa; second, how large the current pre-AIDS HIV epidemic might be; and, finally, what might be the epidemic's growth rate and future toll.

In 1989 the pair published a study that predicted that a typical East or Central African country already in the grips of a severe AIDS epidemic could expect by 1991 to have HIV infection in one out of every five of its citizens.

"That's lowball," Chin said. "It's the high-end estimate based on an overall conservative set of assumptions. It could be a lot worse. Our most conservative estimate is that there will be 575,000 new AIDS cases in Africa in 1991, for a cumulative total of more than 800,000."

Sitting at Chin's side, Mann listened attentively, then said with a heavy voice that the 1990s would be far worse.

"I would like to be optimistic," Mann said, "but I think we must be realistic. Not until 1985 did the message really come home that AIDS was a global problem. In retrospect, probably historians will say it took too long. We are consistently faced with situations where the reality far exceeds our grasp. It's legitimate to ask, 'Are we able to see clearly enough? Or, when we look into the future, is the horror of it all simply too much even for us to confront?' "

But by 1990 Chin's estimates were even grimmer. He was saying that 8 million to 10 million were infected, perhaps 5 million of them in Africa. It would prove the first of many upward revisions.

New WHO Director General Brings Changes

By the time WHO's July 1990 revised forecast was released, Mann and much of his GPA staff were gone. They had lost a power struggle within the Geneva-based organization and Mann had developed a contentious relationship with the new WHO director-general, Hiroshi Nakajima. Mann's enemies within WHO were legion: all those months of greening with envy over the upstart American's meteoric rise finally paid off.

Japanese physician Nakajima, who had headed WHO's Asian regional office during the period when multidrug-resistant malaria spread across the southern region, was clearly uncomfortable with Mann's very public persona and high-profile AIDS program. He shared the views of those who had long whispered derisive comments about the GPA in the WHO hallways. Nakajima felt that disease programs should be managed in accordance with established WHO protocol. It was a reasonable expectation, except for one key point: established protocol did not provide for the contingencies presented by a rapidly expanding worldwide epidemic.

In Mann's stead, Nakajima placed another American physician, Michael Merson. For most of his professional life Merson had worked for WHO in Geneva, managing programs for respiratory and diarrheal diseases. Merson understood WHO protocol.

In Merson's first six months heading GPA, the program upwardly revised its estimates of the size of the global pandemic three times. By September 1990 the official WHO estimate of the cumulative number of AIDS cases was 1.2 million, 400,000 of which were infants and small children—90 percent of whom were in sub-Saharan Africa. And the new WHO year 2000 projection was for 25 million to 30 million HIV infections worldwide.

With concern mounting about the Thirdworldization that AIDS might bring upon Africa, Belgian virologist Peter Piot teamed up with Mead Over to do a systematic analysis of the relative cost of HIV compared to other, better-understood diseases. After carefully computing the per capita burden in terms of productive healthy years of life lost, Piot and Over concluded that the direct costs of treating HIV disease, even in the absence of AZT and other expensive drugs widely available in North America and Western Europe, far outstripped those of any other common ailment in Africa.

The impact was already being felt keenly in some sub-Saharan countries. Malawi's entire health care system, for example, was in genuine peril of collapse under the burden of HIV, and the nation's public-health leadership in 1990 issued desperate pleas to WHO, the World Bank, the U.S. Agency for International Development and other Western organizations for funds.

Even as Africa's leaders began to absorb the direct economic implications of the WHO and World Bank AIDS studies, critics were emerging who charged that the well-intended analyses grossly underestimated the epidemic's impact. For example, nurse Eunice Muringo Kiereini, a Kenyan woman who chaired the WHO Regional Nursing/Midwifery Task Force, claimed that the studies failed to consider the special economic roles women and children played in African economies. Ever since the beginning of Africa's mass urbanization, it had been the continent's young men who left the farms and villages in favor of jobs in the cities. Few village women had the option of abandoning their traditional life-styles. As a result, in many parts of Africa, villages were populated by females of all ages, male children, and elderly men, many of whom were too feeble to work. Young men would return to their wives and children periodically, but their lives were elsewhere.

Food Supply Depends on Women

So it was the women and children of Africa who maintained the continent's agricultural economies, Kiereini said.

Though in some parts of Africa women were less valuable than local livestock—as evidenced by prevailing bride-prices and dowries—it was they who raised the continent's futures: its crops and children. When husbands contracted HIV in the cities and passed the virus on to their wives during periodic return visits to the villages, AIDS appeared in rural areas that were completely lacking in health care and social support systems. The affected women continued to plow the soil with their hand hoes, lugging babies on their backs, until their AIDS-devastated bodies collapsed. And with each female death Africa's agricultural productivity declined another, barely perceptible notch. The cumulative burden of these declines, Kiereini warned, could, by the year 2000, be more desperate for some countries than their losses of professional elites. The demise of Africa's female agricultural workers could, she warned, lead to acute food shortages.

Even uninfected, healthy African women were being forced out of productive roles in agricultural sectors by the AIDS epidemic. In most African societies, both traditionally and under modern codified law, women had virtually no basic rights. They were, legally, their husband's property, as surely as were his cows or goats.

If the husband died, his property reverted not to the wife but to his relatives. The crops that the widow had tilled became a new source of prosperity for the in-laws. The widow and children, now landless, often lacking even changes of clothing, had to find a means of survival.

In the short run, the village and overall societal economies experienced little if any impact from this process because the in-laws continued to harvest crops. But as the epidemic expanded, and even those in-laws were infected, Africa faced the creation of an unprecedented rural underclass of desperately impoverished, often starving women and children. Further, it was obvious that eventually the cumulative load of deprived widows would exceed the available labor force of in-law inheritors, causing declines in crop production.

Worse yet, one of the few survival options left to widows—perhaps the only way they could feed their children—was prostitution. So, impoverished by AIDS, the woman would be forced into a life that virtually guaranteed that she, too, would die of the disease.

By 1991 the gender ratio of AIDS in Africa was shifting, reflecting higher infection rates among women. For example, researchers from the University of California at San Francisco studied 19- to 37-year-old women in Kigali, Rwanda. A third of the randomly sampled women were HIV-positive. Even among women previously thought to be at very low risk for HIV because they were monogamous throughout their lives, the infection rate was 20 percent. The same group also showed that many women in Rwanda were dying of AIDS but not being counted in national statistics because their symptoms didn't fit with the male-based WHO definition of the disease. The researchers suggested that the true extent of AIDS in African women might be two to three times the diagnosed numbers.

Josef Decosas, of Canada's International Development Agency, argued that the continent's women were caught in "an epidemiologic and demographic trap" from which they would not be freed without greater social equity. Decosas contended that any hope of slowing Africa's devastating epidemic before it brought financial ruin to much of the continent was inextricably tied to improvement in the status of Africa's women.

Researchers at the UN's Food and Agriculture Organization, based in Rome, tried to calculate the impact AIDS would have on African agricultural production. Their best estimate was that Africa's overall labor force—predominantly women—would be reduced by 25 percent by 2010.

Another factor compounding estimates of the socioeconomic costs of AIDS was the epidemic's continuing geographic expansion. Though every political leader on the continent knew by 1989–90 what caused the disease and which social measures might prevent its spread, agonizingly few took steps to warn their populaces prior to HIV's full-scale emergence in their midst. South Africa, for example, was spared significant HIV emergence until the late 1980s. There is no evidence that the virus existed in the country prior to 1986, and for the first three years it was almost exclusively a disease of gay white men who had traveled in Europe and North America.

By 1989, however, HIV was emerging in South Africa's black population. The microbe found advantages in apartheid (segregation) policies regarding migrant labor: men from throughout the country, as well as nearby Swaziland, Mozambique and Malawi, were granted work permits for jobs in the gold and diamond mines, but were not allowed to bring their wives and children. Living in squalid barracks, the men frequented brothels in the mining towns whenever possible. Each prostitute became an AIDS amplifier.

By 1991 local experts were estimating that as many as 400,000 black South Africans, mostly men, might be HIV-positive. Given that black infection rates were thought to be near zero two years earlier, this represented explosive growth.

Similarly, Ethiopia, which had long been spared the AIDS scourge, witnessed a phenomenal explosion of cases in 1991–93. As late as 1986 the country had no evidence that HIV had emerged within its borders. In February of that year the first AIDS case was diagnosed in Addis Ababa, the nation's capital. By 1992 local experts estimated that more than 800,000 Ethiopians were infected, with the highest rates of infection—nearly 15 percent—seen among military personnel.

Roy Anderson and his team at Imperial College in London predicted that AIDS in 53 African nations—including several north of the Sahara—"would reverse the size of population growth rates over time scales of a few to many decades."

Meanwhile, the U.S. Census Bureau predicted dire upturns in infant and child mortality in several African nations, due both to direct AIDS deaths and to neglect of children orphaned by the deaths of parents who succumbed to the disease. Hard-won improvements in those two key measures of national development were expected to evaporate. By 1994, the bureau said,

Zambia had already experienced a staggering 15 percent increase in infant mortality, compared with 1984, and Malawi, Uganda and Zaire had suffered nearly comparable increases.

"The concept of a war on AIDS with its goal to stop HIV is seriously flawed and should be discarded," Decosas wrote. "Most regions in the world have a well-established epidemic of HIV. This epidemic requires a social response ranging from a review of legislation to a rethinking of the national industrial-development plans. It also urgently requires new programs, new approaches, and some radical reforms in health care and public health."

4

Asia: Sleeping Giant
of AIDS Epidemic

AFTER TOURING India, Thailand and the Philippines at the request of Speaker of the House Tom Foley (D-Wash.), Representative Jim McDermott, a physician and Democrat from the state of Washington, reached the conclusion that "Asia is the sleeping giant of a worldwide AIDS epidemic." He estimated that as of June 1991 some 1 million Indians were already infected with HIV and in the year 2000 India and Thailand combined would have 12 million infected citizens. McDermott predicted that Asia's epidemic would, within perhaps just five years' time, outstrip that of Africa.

With all the prior warnings, prognostications and clear evidence of the devastation AIDS was inflicting upon Africa, how could the microbe have so overwhelmed Asia? Why hadn't humanity succeeded in preventing HIV's emergence on the continent? As late as the fall of 1989 valid surveys of Thai drug users and prostitutes revealed infection rates below 0.04 percent—seemingly negligible. Yet within a mere 20 months that 0.04

percent infection rate among Chiang Mai prostitutes had soared to more than 70 percent. In just 20 months the virus emerged, spread in an epidemic fashion, and became endemic among key population groups in Thailand. That constituted the most rapid HIV emergence in the history of the global epidemic.

How could this have happened? In retracing the virus's pathway across Asia, scientists and public-health experts gained greater evidence supporting the GPA's earlier theories that human-rights violations, poverty and the behavior of Homo sapiens played crucial roles in the emergence of disease. Indeed, the *only* way to comprehend Thailand's astonishingly rapid HIV emergence was to recognize the intimate coupling of social, political, biological and economic factors.

African history, tragically, repeated itself in Asia. Lessons went unlearned. As had many African societies, most Asian countries initially tried to legislate away the virus by restricting the activities and movement of potential carriers. When that appeared to fail, governments simply refused to acknowledge the virus in their midst, penalizing physicians and experts who raised public alarm about AIDS. Official AIDS figures reported to WHO reflected attempts by most governments to downplay the impact of AIDS.

During the last weeks of 1987 a meeting on AIDS in Asia was convened in Manila, capital of the Philippines, under the partial sponsorship of WHO. Few cases of the disease had, at that point, surfaced in any Asian nation except one, and that country was populated predominantly by Caucasians: Australia. Though Australia was geographically in the Pacific Rim, most Asians considered the country, and its epidemic, European. But Dr. John Dwyer, the avuncular director of AIDS research at the University of South Wales in Sydney, did his best to convince those in attendance at the Manila conference that the pandemic was coming, and it would hit Asia not in the manner of its attack upon Europe but as it had in Africa.

Dwyer pointedly reminded his colleagues that incidences of syphilis, gonorrhea and other sexually transmitted diseases were rapidly rising throughout Asia; that female prostitution was rampant in almost all of the continent's sprawling centers, and male prostitution in several cities; that opium smokers were abandoning that drug and their pipes in favor of heroin and syringes; and that many parts of Asia were suffering levels of poverty and malnutrition comparable to those seen in Africa.

AIDS Takes Indians by Surprise

India's first AIDS cases included recipients of contaminated U.S. blood products manufactured by Cutter Biological, a California-based company, and of anti-RhD vaccines made by Bharat Serums and Vaccine, Ltd., an Indian firm.

During 1985–89 the Indian Council of Medical Research tested more than 2 million people, finding 764 who carried the virus; half of them were female prostitutes. By the end of 1989 the infection rate was soaring. A Bombay survey revealed that 4.9 percent of the city's female prostitutes were infected. As evidence of HIV's presence in India mounted, proposed legislation outlawing sexual intercourse with foreigners was introduced into the Maharashtra state legislature. Though it was defeated, the proposed law reflected a strong mood at that time in Indian society.

So poor were educational efforts that a 1989 survey of a sampling of India's AIDS patients revealed that even they hadn't heard of the disease. Only 4 percent professed to have heard of AIDS before contracting it; most, long after their diagnosis, still had no idea what the disease was. An important factor contributing to ignorance was illiteracy—94 percent of those who were interviewed were unable to read the few AIDS brochures or news articles that were published in India.

By mid-1990 the infection rate among Bombay's prostitutes had risen to 10 percent and 5.6 of every 1,000 blood donors in the city carried the virus. The director of the Indian Medical Research Council, Dr. A. S. Paintal, estimated that Bombay's infection rates had reached such proportions that every day 100,000 sexual acts were performed with HIV-positive female prostitutes. One Bombay STD (sexually transmitted disease) clinic was finding infection rates among prostitutes of 40 percent.

At the same time, blood-donor infection rates rose to 1 percent, and India saw its first cases of HIV involving injecting drug users. Sixty-two heroin users in Manipur were cited in government notices in April 1990. Concern about the blood supply grew when a government survey uncovered 510 HIV-positive blood donors in the state of Gujerat. Among them, 430 were "professional donors," individuals so poor that they subsisted off the meager funds earned by regularly selling their blood. Despite such clear evidence of the microbe's presence in the national blood supply, by the Indian government's admission less than 5 percent of all commercial blood was screened for HIV in 1991. That figure wouldn't budge much in 1992.

Data on HIV infection rates grossly underestimated India's crisis because most high-risk individuals were by 1991 actively avoiding testing. Their reluctance stemmed from widespread knowledge that in Manipur some 100 HIV-positive people were placed in permanent seclusion, chained to their beds, and barred from further social interaction. That drove other potentially infected people underground, away from the public-health system.

One group that was able to penetrate the mistrust was the government's cholera program, which enjoyed widespread respect among India's poor. Their 1991 survey in Manipur revealed that an astonishing 80 percent of heroin injectors were HIV-positive.

The microbe had been handed another bit of good fortune. Beginning around 1987, when Burma, once the richest nation in Southeast Asia, was given the World Bank's least-developed-country status, the traditional opium trade was transformed into a heroin market. It was no longer necessary to ship raw opium paste to Marseilles, France, or other European locales for processing into heroin, thus reducing Burmese profits. But with the shift in opiate processing, heroin was suddenly available for local consumption. Within the so-called Golden Triangle—Burma, southern China and Laos—opium, and now heroin, production outstripped the 1960s market share held by Turkey and Afghanistan.

In Manipur, which borders Burma, the sudden availability of the far more powerful heroin drew opium users like bees to honey. Needles, however, were in short supply.

HIV appeared in Manipur riding the crest of the heroin wave. Former opium smokers clumsily experimented with tourniquets, cookers and syringes, clustering in groups to share not only the knowledge of how to get high but the equipment with which to do so. In less than 16 months, opiate users went from less than 10 percent heroin injectors with under 1 percent HIV seroprevalence to more than 95 percent heroin addicts, mainlining the purest and most powerful smack (heroin) in the world. And 80 percent of them had within that time also mainlined HIV.

Stunned by the rapidity of HIV's march across India, WHO mustered $20 million and the World Bank $100 million for the most aggressively funded AIDS-education campaign ever planned. But from the start the effort seemed doomed, as political leaders throughout India failed to lend their support, some states refused to participate, and allegations of impropriety, even embezzlement, buzzed about the health system. For example, reluctant to face the political flak that would shower down from all over India's business community if the foreign-aid millions were spent outside the country, the government purchased more than a billion defective condoms from a local manufacturer and raised prices on quality imported products.

AIDS Fells Thais

If India's epidemic was racing, Thailand's was moving at supersonic speed. Thai Ministry of Health studies showed that HIV-1 infection rates in nearly every sector of society were well below 2.5 percent in 1989. Eighteen months later double-digit infection rates were the norm all over the country.

Something particularly strange and troublesome happened in Thailand: two separate lineages of HIV-1 emerged, each exploiting entirely different population groups. Among Bangkok heroin injectors there appeared a B-class virus that looked genetically like a typical American HIV. But a very different HIV emerged in Thailand's prostitute and hetero-sexual populations, one that closely resembled a virulent virus seen in Uganda. The two strains moved on separate paths in Thailand, and as of 1993 there was no evidence of cross-mixing of their genetic material.

So Thailand, biologically speaking, had two separate epidemics, both of which grew at unprecedented rates.

The Thai situation demonstrated the folly of dismissing the threat of an emerging microbe merely on the basis of initially small numbers of cases. And it showed, once again, the links between human rights and the emergence of microbes new to a particular society. In the beginning of its epidemic, the Thai government took many of the toughest steps advocated by hard-liners elsewhere in the world. A special HIV-quarantine unit was established in Lard Yao Prison in Bangkok. When, by June 1989, tests indicated that up to 44 percent of the female prostitutes in Chiang Mai were HIV-positive, the government issued decrees in an attempt to crack down on the brothels. As rates of infection soared among heroin addicts, the government ordered Thai police to come down hard on the drug trade and narcotics injectors. Infected foreigners were deported.

Thailand also took positive steps that drew praise from WHO, including establishing the first national HIV sentinel surveillance program in the developing world. By carefully and continuously monitoring levels of HIV infection in key sub-populations of Thai society, the Ministry of Health kept close tabs on the nation's burgeoning epidemic. It may well have been the best-documented HIV emergence in any society in the world.

Despite these efforts the virus spread at record speed throughout the Southeast Asian nation, primarily via its enormous sex industry. As word of the new plague spread, few Thais took steps to protect themselves. Denial, Thai health official Dr. Chai Podhista said in 1992, was the number one problem.

"We have an expression in Thailand," Podhista explained. "It goes, 'If you don't see the body in the coffin, you don't shed a tear.' Rapid spread of the virus is possible—is ignored—because there hasn't yet been mass death. And there won't be for a few years. Hundreds of thousands of people are all getting infected at once, in a clandestine epidemic. Years from now when they all get AIDS, the entire Thai society will go into a state of shock."

At the most crucial moment in its emergence into Thai society, HIV was handed a social gift: human chaos. In February 1991 there was a coup in Thailand, bringing a military junta to power. AIDS programs came to a grinding halt; the flow of nearly all foreign aid, including monies earmarked for HIV control, stopped abruptly. AIDS programs generally fell apart, and the military regime responded to the HIV threat with the sorts of repressive actions that typify juntas: conducting raids on brothels, shutting down those that failed to provide adequate bribes, and rounding up children, alleged slaves and foreign men and women working in the houses of prostitution.

As was the case in Burma and India, the Golden Triangle heroin connection was having an effect on promoting HIV emergence in southern China. Though the government denied it, China had serious heroin, prostitution and sexually transmitted disease incidences that were readily apparent to even casual observers as early as 1987. The most severe problem was in China's southern Yunnan province, which shared borders with Laos and Burma and had long been an opium center. Yunnan narcotics traffickers, like their counterparts in Burma, had learned how to process opium into heroin. By 1991 heroin was in ready supply in Yunnan; syringes were not. By 1993 WHO was estimating that up to a third of Yunnan heroin users were infected.

Less than a year later WHO announced that heroin was driving a terrible HIV epidemic in Ho Chi Minh City, Vietnam. Among heroin users the HIV rate climbed from less than 2 percent to more than 30 percent in about nine months' time.

As had been the case with Africa's AIDS epidemic, Asia watchers wondered aloud whether the pandemic might reverse the region's famed "Economic Miracle," causing a Thirdworld-

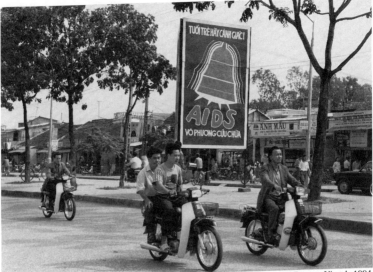

Anti-AIDS propaganda on a main street of Hanoi, the Vietnamese capital, in 1994.

ization effect. If local epidemics continued to expand at their breathtaking 1989–93 rates, Asia could be expected to overtake Africa in HIV numbers before the turn of the century. And ironically, the fiscal cost to Asia would be greater precisely because the continent's economy had boomed so impressively during the 1980s. With greater prosperity came higher costs. The dollar value of productive capacity lost due to worker illness and death was greater in Asia (compared with Africa) simply because there was a larger highly skilled labor force and incomes across-the-board were higher. Direct medical costs were higher as well, because of the availability of more sophisticated—and costly—health care systems.

Still, it seemed at first glance unimaginable that AIDS could make a dent in Asia's economic boom. Only a handful of countries (the Philippines, Papua New Guinea, Burma and Cambodia) experienced negative GNP growth during the 1980s, and many Asian countries had growth rates that were five to seven times greater than those of the United States and Switzerland.

Like Africa, however, much of Asia was simultaneously undergoing other disease emergences that could be expected to compound or synergize with HIV/AIDS. These included dengue, hepatitis (A, B, C, D and E), multiply drug-resistant malaria, tuberculosis, drug-resistant cholera, and virtually every known sexually transmissible microbe. Though no one knew how to calculate the additive or multiplicative economic impacts the interlocking epidemics might have, it was clear, biologically and epidemiologically speaking, that interconnections existed.

There was a clear consensus in international public-health circles by 1993 that the pandemic would, at the very least, exert a Thirdworldization effect upon the health care systems, tourist industries, and government-funded social-service sectors of hard-hit countries. Worst-case scenarios forecast sharp declines in both agricultural and industrial productivity with resultant declines in gross domestic products. The UN Development Program and the Asian Development Bank predicted in late 1993 that the HIV epidemic would increase general levels of poverty and, by the year 2000, cause local famines in key areas.

Such dire economic forecasts, whether they concerned the projected impact of AIDS on Africa, Asia, or Latin America, were always intended to draw the attention of wealthy donor states. The nations of North America, Western Europe, and, to a lesser degree, Japan and the former Soviet Union had always been forthcoming with cash when a crisis struck, even if the quantities were more symbolic than substantial. If the cash was offered at interest, Africa and Latin America might cringe, but Asia had an excellent debt-repayment record.

5

Threats to Health
in the Industrialized World

THROUGHOUT THE WORLD hope for a global AIDS bailout rose as Berliners clawed away at the wall that had physically divided their city for three decades. What began with dockworkers in Gdansk, Poland, in the early 1980s, built slowly for years in pockets of antiauthoritarian resistance that spanned from Prague, Czechoslovakia, to Riga, Latvia, from Vladivostok, Russia, to Berlin, Germany. Once the Berlin Wall fell there was no turning back: the ideal and reality of communism were dead. And with the end of communism came capitalist dominance and Western victory in the cold war. Threat of global thermonuclear annihilation suddenly seemed quite remote. Politicians all over the world spoke of a "peace dividend." And suddenly the world had surplus cash, they claimed, and long-neglected social programs could now be subsidized. For a few months in history, it seemed, people around the world were remarkably optimistic.

But no peace dividend appeared. People craned their necks

looking for it, soon spotting a shadow emerging on the horizon. Excitement yielded to despair and frustration as they recognized the shadowy dividend for what it was: international recession.

After all the celebrations and dancing in the streets of Prague and Berlin settled down, the West got a good, hard look at what lay behind the Berlin Wall, inside the long-sequestered world of communism. And they discovered that Stalinists from Uzbekistan to the Baltics had been juggling the books for decades. The East was broke.

Worse yet, its populations, which had long had nearly every aspect of their lives controlled by the state, were ill prepared to build strong civic societies. With their economies in a shambles, cynicism quickly overcame the brief sensation of elation for most Europeans.

Overnight the former cold-war multitrillion-dollar spending became a latter-day Marshall Plan for reconstruction of the ex-Communist world. Ten billion dollars shifted from coffers in Bonn, Germany, to national bank vaults in Moscow, Russia, in a single day. And that was just one of many West-to-East transfers.

Not only was there no peace dividend, there was newfound, long-term structural agony. Even the booming Asian economies felt the pain as demand for autos, electronics, and consumer goods dropped in Europe and North America.

While much of the world watched the demolition of the Berlin Wall during the fall of 1989 with astonishment and elation, AIDS activist Hans Seyfarth-Hermann dashed about Checkpoint Charlie, gateway to West Berlin, tossing condoms at the crowds of East Germans as they poured through. The bewildered East Germans snapped the packets out of the air and examined what looked like matchbook covers. They read this brightly colored inscription: "You will see many tantalizing things during your visit to West Berlin. Enjoy yourself, but remember, we have AIDS."

Inside each putative matchbook was a latex condom. Political openness, it appeared, could carry a price tag. If it was true, as the old Stalinist leaders claimed, that AIDS hadn't made its way yet into most of Eastern Europe, the fall of the Berlin Wall would surely put an end to the political barriers that had allegedly kept the microbe at bay.

HIV would also ride Europe's new heroin trail. Opening up the formerly secluded states rang bells of opportunity for organized criminal elements on both sides of the former wall. Poland, in particular, would become both a center for a locally produced opiate called *kompot* and a transfer point for pure heroin imported from other parts of the world and destined for distribution in Central Europe.

The first serious emergences of HIV in Eastern Europe were not via either prostitution or heroin injection, however. Rather, they came by means that reflected the tragic state of medicine in much of the Communist bloc.

1988 Saw AIDS Emergence in Russia

Though there had been isolated AIDS cases in Russia for at least four years, HIV really emerged during the early spring of 1988 in Elista, capital of the Kalmyk Republic, located on the Caspian Sea. A baby languished on the pediatric ward of the town's hospital, suffering every imaginable ailment. Doctors were stumped, unable to reach a diagnosis, until one suggested sending blood samples from the infant to Valentin Pokrovsky, a virologist doing AIDS research in Moscow. Pokrovsky confirmed that the child was infected with HIV.

The child's father, it turned out, had visited the Congo in 1981, where he apparently was exposed to HIV. He passed the virus sexually to his wife, who, in turn, transmitted HIV to the child.

It was tantamount to treason to publicly acknowledge shortages of vital goods during the regime of Joseph Stalin (1924–53), and 40 years after the dictator's death many Soviet citizens remained reluctant to step outside normal bureaucratic channels in order to draw attention to production deficiencies. In 1988, however, prior to news from Elista, U.S.S.R. Minister of Health Alexander Kondrusev publicly decried the country's sorry state of medical supplies. In particular, he warned that the nation needed to use 3 billion syringes per year, but was only manufacturing 30 million annually, and importing none. Simple mathematics indicated, then, that the average syringe was being used 100 times. Kondrusev warned that this syringe shortage could spell disaster.

He would soon prove remarkably prescient.

The AIDS baby at the Elista hospital was treated by staff who used the same syringes to withdraw blood samples from and administer drugs to all the babies on the neonatal ward. For more than three months the nurses unknowingly injected HIV into all of the babies and, in a few cases, their mothers.

As the numbers of AIDS babies mounted, the overwhelmed Elista doctors ordered some of the infants shipped to a hospital in Volgograd. And again, the medical staff reused syringes over and over, soon having infected nearly every child on the Volgograd baby ward.

The incidents were kept quiet until early 1989 when a Russian trade union newspaper, *Trud,* broke the story. According to *Trud,* Health Minister Kondrusev had grossly underestimated the enormity of the gap in the Soviet Union between the number of injection procedures of one kind or another that were performed by health providers and the annual production rate of sterile syringes. While leaders in Moscow received single-use sterile injections, the masses living in outlying areas relied on hospitals that suffered permanent supply shortages. So in Elista and Volgograd, for example, health care workers had little choice but to reuse syringes 400 or 500 times, occasionally honing the needles on a whetstone so that they would still pierce skin.

It was horribly reminiscent of the events in Yambuku Hospital in 1976, where Belgian nuns used a handful of syringes hundreds of times per week, unwittingly spreading the deadly Ebola virus. That, however, occurred in a remote, impoverished region of Central Africa; the Soviet Union was, allegedly, part of the advanced industrial world.

But Soviet leaders were preoccupied with far more-pressing

issues than supplies of syringes. The country was literally falling apart. Food shortages, riots, separatist uprisings, political instability and a face-off between the hero of *glasnost* (openness), Mikhail S. Gorbachev (1985–91), and upstart leader (now president) Boris S. Yeltsin monopolized national attention. By 1991 the Soviet Union no longer existed. By 1993 two major coup attempts had threatened the stability of the Russian Republic, and insurrections had occurred inside most of the former Soviet socialist states.

Social Breakdown Promotes Spread of Disease

AIDS was overshadowed by history. And the microbe spread, unfettered by any serious efforts on the part of human beings to limit its modes of transmission. Prostitution and drug abuse stepped into the economic vacuum of social restructuring. Criminal elements gained control of many foreign-trade sectors, and syringes remained in short supply.

By late 1993 the microbial situation was clearly out of control. Before the Berlin Wall fell, Russia's syphilis rate was 4.3 cases per 100,000 people annually. Amid the national chaos, health officials said they were witnessing a syphilis epidemic. In St. Petersburg, for example, the incidence of syphilis increased eightfold between 1989 and 1993, with most of the newly infected individuals young, destitute female prostitutes. In the same city the incidence of gonorrhea among teenagers had soared 150 percent by 1993, as compared with 1976 levels. And in the same subpopulation, syphilis incidence was up 400 percent.

Dr. Nikolai Chaika, of the St. Petersburg Pasteur Institute, announced that all Russian disease data, including numbers of HIV/AIDS cases, were unreliable due to the "complete collapse of Russian medicine." The social fabric of Russian society was unraveling, he said, and people were turning to behaviors that virtually guaranteed the spread of disease.

Thirdworldization had set in. In the summer of 1992 cholera outbreaks were reported in Makhachkala, Nizhny Novgorod, Krasnodar, Naberezhnye Nizhny and Moscow. The Tass news agency reported an outbreak of anthrax among peasants in the Altai region and typhoid fever in Volgodonsk. Even a case of bubonic plague was reported from Kazakhstan.

Separate European Community studies of Russian health revealed that tuberculosis rates were climbing sharply. In Siberia in 1990 there was a TB incidence of 43 cases per 100,000 people (as measured by positive sputum). By 1993 that ratio had more than doubled, to 94:100,000. Over the same period, Moscow's TB rate jumped from 27:100,000 to 50:100,000. The principal cause of the escalation was said to be the lack of foreign exchange with which to purchase European- and American-made antituberculosis drugs; without treatment an ever-expanding pool of contagious individuals was spreading the disease to others.

Perhaps the most striking examples of Russian Thirdworldization were the 1993 outbreaks of diphtheria in St. Petersburg and Moscow.

A hallmark of the old Soviet Union had been its tremendous success in universal vaccination and resultant declines in the incidence of former scourges such as measles, whooping cough, polio and diphtheria. By 1976 the numbers of diphtheria cases diagnosed in the U.S.S.R. approached zero.

But in 1990 diphtheria reemerged in Russia, with 1,211 cases reported from St. Petersburg, Kaliningrad, Orlovskaya and Moscow. The epidemic took off, with reported cases and geographic spread increasing steadily well into 1994. In 1991 nearly 1,900 diphtheria cases and 80 deaths were reported in Russia. Though the bacterial disease could be treated with antibiotics, deaths occurred due to the sorry state of the nation's health care systems.

AIDS in the United States Strains 'Safety Net'

There was no need to search behind the Iron Curtain, the Bamboo Curtain, or below the Sahara to witness microbial exploitation of Thirdworldization. The process was occurring during the 1980s and the early 1990s inside the wealthy nations of North America and Western Europe.

Despite the AIDS epidemic, most of the public-health community, which was not involved in infectious diseases work, remained optimistic during the 1980s. So much so that health became a matter of personal responsibility. Health economists tallied up the costs of diseases that were preventable through diet, exercise, cessation of tobacco or illicit drug use, elimination of alcoholism and the like, reaching the conclusion that personal health decisions were no longer the exclusive purview of individual choice. Smokers, they concluded, cost the rest of society billions of dollars. So did alcoholics. And fat people.

"The cost of sloth, gluttony, alcoholic intemperance, reckless driving, sexual frenzy and smoking is now a national and not an individual responsibility," wrote Dr. John Knowles, president of the Rockefeller Foundation. "This is justified as individual freedom—but one man's freedom in health is another man's shackle in taxes and insurance premiums. I believe that a right to health should be replaced by the idea of an individual moral obligation to preserve one's own health—a public duty, if you will."

Public-health advocates warned, however, that it was exceedingly unfair, and unrealistic, to hold poor Americans responsible for their health—to condemn them, as it seemed Knowles did, for their inability to afford ideal foods, membership in exercise clubs, and temperance in all sexual and intoxicant affairs. Further, they warned that the medical triumphs that had sparked such rosy calls for personal responsibility were fleeting. In the face of rising poverty, they said, the old scourges would return.

It wasn't necessary to go to Africa to see AIDS orphans or whole families buried side by side. New York City alone would have more than 30,000 AIDS orphans by the end of 1994, Newark, New Jersey, over 10,000. The U.S. Department of Health and Human Services predicted that there would be 60,000 AIDS orphans in the country by the year 2000. Just as AIDS was exhausting the extended-family networks in much of Africa, so it was taxing the social-support systems in America's poorest communities.

With every passing year in America's AIDS epidemic, the impact upon the nation's poorest urban areas grew even more severe. It compounded the effects of other plights—homelessness, drug abuse, alcoholism, high infant mortality, syphilis, gonorrhea, violence—all of which conspired to increase levels of desperation where dreams of urban renewal had once existed.

As the virus found its way into communities of poverty, the burden on urban public hospitals was critical. Unlike Canada and most of Western Europe, the United States had no system of national health care. By 1990 an estimated 37 million Americans were without any form of either public or private health insurance. Too rich to qualify for government-supported health care, which was intended only for the elderly and the indigent, but too poor to purchase private insurance, millions of Americans simply prayed that they wouldn't fall ill. Another 43 million Americans were either chronically uninsured or under-insured, possessing such minimal coverage that the family could be bankrupted by the required deductible and copayments in the event of serious illness.

AIDS Overwhelms Public Hospital System

Any disease that hit poor urban Americans disproportionately would tax the public hospital system. But AIDS, which was particularly costly and labor-intensive to treat, threatened to be the straw that broke the already weakened back of the system.

"We are fighting a war here," declared Dr. Emilio Carrillo, president of the New York City Health and Hospitals Corporation, which ran the city's network of public medical facilities. "People are sick and dying from AIDS, tuberculosis is rampant, malnutrition, drug addiction and other diseases resulting from poverty are also at epidemic levels, while at every level of government, city, state and federal, the health care system is facing cutbacks. Only the number of sick people and people in need of basic health care is not being cut back. Among them there have been no reductions, no downsizing. They are still coming in to us for treatment."

A 1990 survey of 100 of the nation's largest public hospitals (conducted by the National Association of Public Hospitals) revealed worsening situations in all American cities and predicted collapse of the "public safety net" offered by the system. A microbe that had emerged in America only a decade earlier was threatening to topple the system.

In 1993 the New York City Heath Department announced that life expectancy for men in the city had *declined,* for the first time since World War II, from a 1981 level of 68.9 years to a 1991 level of 68.6 years. This occurred even though outside New York City life expectancies for men in the state had *risen* during that time from 71.5 years to 73.4 years. Though rising homicide rates played a role, city officials credited AIDS with the bulk of that downward shift. By 1987 AIDS was already the leading cause of premature death for New York City men of all races and classes; by 1988 it was the number one cause for African-American women as well.

Well before AIDS was claiming significant numbers of Americans, Harlem Hospital chief of surgery Dr. Harold Freeman calculated that men growing up in Bangladesh had a better chance of surviving to their 65th birthday than did African-American men in Harlem, the Bronx, or Brooklyn. Again, violence played a significant role in the equation, but it was not critical to why a population of hundreds of thousands of men living in the wealthiest nation on earth were living shorter lives than their counterparts in one of the planet's poorest Third World nations. Average life expectancy for Harlem's African-American men born between 1950 and 1970 was just 49 years. Freeman indicted disease, poverty and inequitable access to medical care as the primary factors responsible for the alarming death rate among African-American men.

Well before a new tuberculosis epidemic struck several U.S. cities, the warning signs were there for all to see: rising homelessness, fiscal reductions in social services, complacency in the public-health sector, rampant drug abuse and increases in a number of other infectious diseases. The emergence of novel strains of multiply drug-resistant TB came amid a host of clangs, whistles and bells that should have served as ample warning to humanity. But the warning fell on unhearing ears.

Some of the microbial impact of this urban Thirdworldization might have been controllable had the U.S. public-health system been vigilant. But at all tiers, from the grass roots to the federal level, the system was by the mid-1980s in a very sorry state. Complacent after decades of perceived victories over the microbes, positioned as the runt sibling to curative medicine and fiscally pared to the bone by successive rounds of budget cuts in all layers of government, public health in 1990 was a mere shadow of its former self.

An Institute of Medicine investigation determined that public-health and disease-control efforts in the United States were in a shambles. Key problems included "a lack of agreement about the public-health mission" between various sectors of government and research; a clear failure of public-health advocates to participate in "the dynamics of American politics"; lack of cooperation between medicine and public health; inadequate training and leadership; and severe funding deficiencies at all levels.

Conclusion

U LTIMATELY, humanity will have to change its perspective on its place in Earth's ecology if the species hopes to stave off or survive the next plague. Rapid globalization of human niches requires that human beings everywhere on the planet go beyond viewing their neighborhoods, provinces, countries, or hemispheres as the sum total of their personal ecospheres. Microbes, and their vectors, recognize none of the artificial boundaries erected by human beings. Theirs is the world of natural limitations: temperature, pH, ultraviolet light, the presence of vulnerable hosts and mobile vectors.

In the microbial world, warfare is a constant. The survival of most organisms necessitates the demise of others. Yeasts secrete antibiotics to ward off attacking bacteria. Viruses invade the bacteria and commandeer their genetic machinery to viral advantage.

A glimpse into the microbial world, aided by powers of exponential magnification, reveals a frantic, angry place, a colorless, high-speed pushing-and-shoving match that makes the lunch-hour sidewalk traffic of Tokyo seem positively poky. If microbes had elbows, one imagines they would forever be jabbing neighbors in an endless battle for biological turf.

Yet there are times of extraordinary collectivity in the microbial world, when the elbowing yields to combating a shared enemy. Swapping genes to counter an antibiotic threat or secreting a beneficial chemical inside a useful host to allow continued parasitic comfort is illustrative of this microscopic coincidence.

The Mighty Microbe

An individual microbe's world—its ecological milieu—is limited only by the organism's mobility and its ability to tolerate various ranges of temperature, sunlight, oxygen, acidity or alkalinity and other factors in its soupy existence. Wherever there may be an ideal soup for a microbe, it will eagerly take hold, immediately joining in the local microbial pushing and shoving. Whether transported to fresh soup by its own micromotor and flagella or with the external assistance of wind, human intercourse, flea, or an iota of dust makes little difference provided the soup in which the organism lands is minimally hostile and maximally comfortable.

The planet is nothing but a crazy quilt of microsoups scattered all over its 196,938,800-square-mile surface.

We, as individuals, can't see them, or sense their presence in any useful manner. The most sophisticated of their species have the ability to outwit or manipulate the one microbial sensing system Homo sapiens possess: our immune systems. By sheer force of numbers they overwhelm us. And they are evolving far more rapidly than Homo sapiens, adapting to changes in their environments by mutating, undergoing high-speed natural selection, or drawing plasmids and transposons from the vast mobile genetic lending library in their environments.

Further, every microscopic pathogen is a parasite that survives by feeding off a higher organism. The parasites are themselves victims of parasitism. Like a Russian wooden doll-within-a-doll, the intestinal worm is infected with bacteria, which are infected with tiny phage viruses. The whale has a gut

68

full of algae, which are infected with *Vibrio cholerae*. Each microparasite is another rivet in the Global Village airplane. Interlocked in sublimely complicated networks of webbed systems, they constantly adapt and change. Every individual alteration can change an entire system; each systemic shift can propel an interlaced network in a radical new direction.

In this fluid complexity human beings stomp about with swagger, elbowing their way without concern into one ecosphere after another. The human race seems equally complacent about blazing a path into a rain forest with bulldozers and arson or using an antibiotic "scorched earth" policy to chase unwanted microbes across the duodenum. In both macroecology and microecology, human beings appear, as Harvard's Dick Levins put it, "utterly incapable of embracing complexity."

Only by appreciating the fine nuances in their ecologies can human beings hope to understand how their actions, on the macro level, affect their micro competitors and predators.

Time is short.

As the Homo sapiens population swells, surging past the 6 billion mark at the millennium, the opportunities for pathogenic microbes multiply. If, as some have predicted, 100 million of those people might then be infected with HIV, the microbes will have an enormous pool of walking immune-deficient petri dishes in which to thrive, swap genes and undergo endless evolutionary experiments.

"We are in an eternal competition. We have beaten out virtually every other species to the point where we may now talk about protecting our former predators," Joshua Lederberg told a 1994 Manhattan gathering of investment bankers. "But we're not alone at the top of the food chain."

Our microbe predators are adapting, changing, evolving, he warned. "And any more rapid change would be at the cost of human devastation."

The human world was a very optimistic place on September 12, 1978, when over 130 ministers of health at a WHO convention in the U.S.S.R. signed the Declaration of Alma-Ata. By the year 2000 all of humanity was supposed to be immunized against most infectious diseases, basic health care was to be available to every man, woman and child regardless of their economic class, race, religion, or place of birth.

But as the world approaches the millennium, it seems, from the microbes' point of view, as if the entire planet, occupied by nearly 6 billion mostly impoverished Homo sapiens, is like the city of Rome in 5 B.C.

"The world really is just one village. Our tolerance of disease in any place in the world is at our own peril," Lederberg said. "Are we better off today than we were a century ago? In most respects, we're worse off. We have been neglectful of the microbes, and that is a recurring theme that is coming back to haunt us."

In the end, it seems that American journalist I. F. Stone was right when he said, "Either we learn to live together or we die together."

While the human race battles itself, fighting over ever more crowded turf and scarcer resources, the advantage moves to the microbes' court. They are our predators and they will be victorious if we, Homo sapiens, do not learn how to live in a rational global village that affords the microbes few opportunities.

It's either that or we brace ourselves for the coming plague.

Talking It Over
A Note for Students and Discussion Groups

This issue of the HEADLINE SERIES, like its predecessors, is published for every serious reader, specialized or not, who takes an interest in the subject. Many of our readers will be in classrooms, seminars or community discussion groups. Particularly with them in mind, we present below some discussion questions—suggested as a starting point only—and references for further reading.

Discussion Questions

The international effort to eradicate smallpox crossed political, national, cultural, racial and religious boundaries and often took on military overtones. Would such an effort succeed today? What sort of crisis could generate similar support?

Why did the international campaign against smallpox succeed but the effort to eradicate malaria fail?

What makes the AIDS epidemic different from other epidemics? Why did neither the smallpox nor malaria eradication campaign serve as a model for a global response to AIDS?

What lessons have societies learned from dealing with AIDS that can be applied to combating future disease epidemics?

Reading List

Carson, Rachel, *Silent Spring.* Boston, Houghton Mifflin, 1987.

Garrett, Laurie, "The Return of Infectious Disease." *Foreign Affairs,* Jan./Feb. 1996.

Lappé, M., *Germs That Won't Die.* Garden City, N.Y., Anchor Press, 1982.

Levy, S. B., *The Antibiotic Paradox.* New York, Plenum Press, 1992.

Gore, Al, *Earth in the Balance.* New York, Houghton Mifflin, 1992.

Mann, Jonathan, Caraballo, Manuel, et al., eds., *The Global Impact of AIDS.* New York, Wiley, 1988.

Morse, S. S., "Controlling Infectious Diseases." *Technology Review,* October 1995.

World Health Organization Press Office, 1211 Geneva 27, Switzerland (Fax 791-0746). Extensive relevant publications include the following: Malaria: Fact Sheet No. 94, Nov. '95; New and Reemerging Infectious Diseases: Fact Sheet No. 97, Nov. '95; *Our Planet, Our Health* (Report to the United Nations Earth Summit, Rio de Janeiro, Brazil, June 1992).